# Practical Record Book for Community Health Nursing

# Practical Record Book for Community Health Nursing

**Manju John**
BSc(N) MSc (N) MA (Sociology & Public Administration)
DN Adm PhD

Principal
SAM College of Nursing
Bhopal, Madhya Pradesh, India

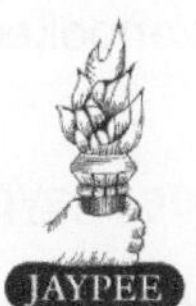


**JAYPEE BROTHERS MEDICAL PUBLISHERS**
*The Health Sciences Publisher*
New Delhi | London

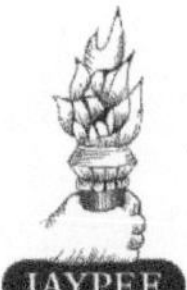

**Jaypee Brothers Medical Publishers (P) Ltd**

**Headquarters**
EMCA House
23/23-B, Ansari Road, Daryaganj
New Delhi 110 002, India
Landline: +91-11-23272143, +91-11-23272703
+91-11-23282021, +91-11-23245672
E-mail: jaypee@jaypeebrothers.com

**Corporate Office**
4838/24, Ansari Road, Daryaganj
New Delhi 110 002, India
Phone: +91-11-43574357
Fax: +91-11-43574314
E-mail: jaypee@jaypeebrothers.com

**Overseas Office**
J.P. Medical Ltd.
83, Victoria Street, London
SW1H 0HW (UK)
Phone: +44-20 3170 8910
E-mail: info@jpmedpub.com

**EU GPSR** Authorised Representative
Logos Europe, 9 rue Nicolas Poussin
17000, La Rochelle, France
Phone: +33 (0) 6 67 93 73 78
E-mail: contact@logoseurope.eu

Website: www.jaypeebrothers.com
Website: www.jaypeedigital.com



**Inquiries for bulk sales may be solicited at:** jaypee@jaypeebrothers.com

***Practical Record Book for Community Health Nursing***

*First Edition*: 2015, *Reprint:* **2025**

ISBN: 978-93-5152-541-7

*Printed in India*

**Dedicated to**

*The revered memory of my husband–*
*Late Mr Shailendra C John*
*who is always in my life;*
*the loving memory of my father–*
*Late Dr YP Masih*
*who taught me always to continue education, humanistic care and*
*be the best teacher in the nursing profession*

# Student's Details

Paste your Photo

Name of the Institution: ______________________________

Nursing Course: ______________________________

Subject: Community Health Nursing

Name of the Candidate: ______________________________

Roll Number: ______________________________

Signature of the External Examiner

Signature of the Internal Examiner

Signature of the Principal

## VISION

- **Practical Record Book for Community Health Nursing**

## MISSION

- I will be of service even in the remotest part of our country.
- I will speak the positive language of young India.
- I will be prompt for patients/clients.
- I will assume responsibilities as a professional and competent nurse.
- I will make independent decision in nursing situation.
- I will protect the rights of patients/clients in the hospital/community nursing.
- I will offer excellence in nursing service.
  (To those abroad, as much as I do to those in India)

## VALUES

We will always respect our clients/patients in hospital,
urban and rural field.
We will always be honest, transparent and ethical.
We will nurture pride in India.

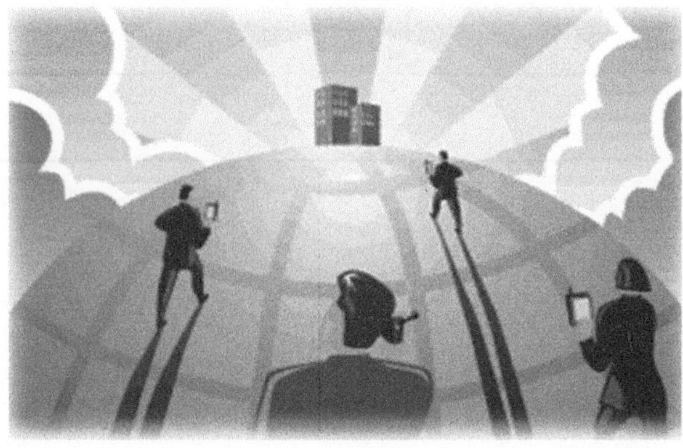

# Preface

*All nursing families are trusted from generation to generation and our real achievement is that one and all nursing candidates become delighted by using 'Practical Record Book for Community Health Nursing'.*

It is the great rays of inspiration, pleasure and satisfaction that are required to prepare *Practical Record Book for Community Health Nursing* for nursing students. Nurses play a crucial role in protecting patient safety and providing quality health care. Nursing professional has been identified as an indispensable entity in the care of the sick, injured and unhealthy; it has further been extended to the health of the community.

The main purpose of this book is to provide knowledge to student nurses posted in community health nursing care settings to fulfill the required field experience as per Indian Nursing Council syllabus.

This book is designed for graduate, postgraduate, general nursing courses and other professional nursing courses. It provides information that is related to community-based field visit areas, surveys and orientation reports, procedures, family folders and various assignments, etc.

It is hoped that this book will help all nursing students and professionals towards rejuvenation thinking in community care with an innovative idea for community health nursing.

**Manju John**

# Acknowledgments

The book *Practical Record book for Community Health Nursing* is based on the course and curricula of the nursing students.

I am greatly indebted and sincerely grateful to the almighty God for showering upon me his blessings. Without Him, this work would not have been possible.

I thank my family members, late Mr Shailendra C John, Prerna John and Akansha John for their unending support, encouragement and patience in helping me during the entire chore of the book work.

My special thanks are due to several people who motivated me in this venture. I thank the teachers for their constant help and support.

I also thank M/s Jaypee Brothers Medical Publishers (P) Ltd, New Delhi, India, for publishing this book and accomplishing the task in a splendid manner.

Lastly, I recommend to nursing students to use this practical record book that supports and guides in a comprehensive manner while achieving competence to practice nursing safely and effectively.

## PROPER USE OF PRACTICAL RECORD BOOK AND ITS IMPORTANCE

1. It gives the identification profile of the student.
2. It is the blueprint of clinical experience.
3. It helps the candidate at the time of interview with the Government and non-Government organizations.
4. It helps the candidate to recall the community field experience within a short duration.
5. It gives the information about subject papers and their theoretical and community field experience hours.
6. It helps the student to remember the basic important formulas and normal values of blood/serum with urine output.
7. This practical experience record book based on the syllabus according to Indian Nursing Council, covers all the community field/PHC/CHC/SC/practical areas according to the course year.
8. This practical book will be helpful in monitoring the community health nursing performances of the students.
9. This practical experience record book will help the faculty members to implement the practical syllabus effectively.
10. Students should make the signature in prescribed areas after doing the procedure under the supervision of nursing tutor/clinical instructor/community health nurse guide.
11. When the student has completed the demonstration and practice, this book should be submitted to the principal and the class teacher for signature about 15 days before exam.
12. No student is allowed to write unnecessary matter in the procedure book.
13. Student should handle practical experience record book safely, keep with brown cover, photo should be fixed in the space provided, and all the necessary information to be filled along the signature of the student.
14. When the students have the repeat practical exams, they should receive signature from both the internal and external examiners in the space provide for repeat.
15. In case of the loss of the practical record book, student can purchase new record book as early as possible and get all the signatures from the teachers and principal; institute is not responsible for completing the record.

# Contents

# SECTION-1

BSc (N) Second (II) Year,
Post Basic BSc (N), MSc (N)

# 1. INTRODUCTION

The community has been described as one of the most fruitful areas for improving the health of the people. It is a fact that social, physical and cultural aspects of the community have a major influence on an individual health status. The social environment is important since social problem and social support are directly related to physical and mental illness. Similarly, physical environment is important since physical problems like air, water and soil pollution lead to various diseases in human beings.

Nurses and all health professionals must actively consider the influence of the community on the health status of the patient. More importantly, nurses need to become involved in influencing the structure and functioning of system within the community. A focus on preserving and promoting health and preventing illness for all people in the community will not only have an impact on the health of the identified client, but will also reach the lives of numerous people who are not in the health care system. So, it is important to review the community once again to get acquainted with its concepts.

## MEANING OF COMMUNITY

The word 'community' is used in a variety of contexts and by the people with different perspectives. The term 'community' suggests a shared pattern of feelings, behaviors and lifestyles together with close and frequent personal relationship with others (little wood, 1985).

The word community has been derived from two Latin words; namely 'com' and 'munis' means to serve. Thus, community means to serve together, it means the community is an organization of human beings framed for the purposes of serving together.

## DEFINITION OF COMMUNITY

'Community is a group of people who live together, who belong together, so that share, not ties or that particular interest, but as a whole set of interests, wide enough and complete enough to include their lives.' He included in 'community' small aggregation, such as villages, and large ones as cities and tribes and nations (McIver).

a. Community is the smallest territorial group that can embrace all aspects of social life (Kingsley Davis)
b. A society that inhabits in a definite geographical area is known as community (MC Manzer)
c. A community may be defined as a permanent local aggregation of people having diversified as well as common interest and served by a constellation of institution (Lumbi).
d. Community is a living population within a limited geographical area carrying on a common interest (Lund Berg).

## AIMS OF COMMUNITY HEALTH NURSING

1. Reduction of risk factors to reduce morbidity and mortality rate.
2. Strengthening self-care activities to promote the health and prevent the occurrence of diseases.
3. Maintain the quality of life to live productive life.
4. Improving standard of living to protect the health against diseases.

## PRINCIPLES OF COMMUNITY HEALTH NURSING

- Provide community services continuation.
- Appraisal and evaluation of services.
- Based on community needs.
- No acceptance of bribe/gift.
- Consider nursing ethics.
- Family as a basic unit.
- Assist family in making decisions related to health.
- Maintain record.
- Job satisfaction.
- No discrimination age, caste, creed, sex.
- Professional IPR.
- Collaboration and coordination.
- Community participation.
- Qualified nursing personnel and continuing education program.
- Create awareness through education.
- Follow-up.
- Involve leaders or influential people.

## OBJECTIVES

- Identify community profile.
- Identify prevalent communicable and non-communicable diseases.
- Diagnose health needs of individual, families and community.
- Plan, provide and evaluate care.
- Participate in School Health Program.
- Participate in National Health Program.
- Organize group for self-help and involve clients in their own health activities.
- Provide family welfare services.
- Council and educate individual, family and community.
- Collect vital statistics.
- Maintain records and reports.

## SKILLS

- Community health survey.
- Community diagnosis.
- Family care: Home adaptation of common procedure.
- Home visit: Bag technique.
- Organize and conduct clinics: Antenatal, postnatal, well baby clinic, camps, etc.
- Screen manage and referrals for.
- High-risk mothers and neonates.
- Accidents and emergencies.
- Illness: Physical and mental.

## ABILITIES

- Conduct delivery at center/home: episiotomy and suturing
- Resuscitate newborn
- School Health Program.
- Screen, manage, and refer children.

- Collaborate with health and allied agencies.
- Train and supervise health workers
- Provide family welfare services: Insertion of IUD.
- Counsel and teach individual, family and community about HIV, TB, diabetes, hypertension mental health, adolescents, elderly's health, physically and mentally challenged individuals, etc.
- Collect and calculate vital health statistics.
- Document and maintain
- Individual, family and administrative records.
- Write reports: Center, Disease, National Health Program/Projects.

## STAFFING PATTERN: COMMUNITY HEALTH CENTER

| Sl. No. | Post | Number |
|---|---|---|
| | *EXISTING CLINICAL MANPOWER* | |
| 1. | General Surgeon | 1 |
| 2. | Physician | 1 |
| 3. | Obstetrician/Gynecologist | 4 |
| 4. | Pediatrician | 1 |
| | *PROPOSED CLINICAL MANPOWER* | |
| 1. | Anesthetist | 1 |
| 2. | Eye surgeon | 1 |
| 3. | Public Health Program Manager | 1 |
| | *EXISTING SUPPORT MANPOWER* | |
| 1. | Nurse – midwife | 7 + 2 |
| 2. | Dresser | 1 |
| 3. | Lab Technician | 1 |
| 4. | Radiographer | 1 |
| 5. | Ward boy/Nursing orderly | 1 |
| 6. | Sweepers | 0 – 1 |
| 7. | Chowkidar | 2 |
| 8. | OPD Attendant | 3 |
| 9. | Statistical Assistant/Data Entry Operator | 5 |
| 10. | OT Attendant | |
| 11. | Registration Clerk | |
| | TOTAL | 21 – 22 + 2 |

## PRIMARY HEALTH CENTER

| Sl. No. | Post | Number |
|---|---|---|
| 1. | Medical Officer | 1 |
| 2. | Pharmacist | 1 |
| 3. | Nurse Midwife | 1 |
| 4. | Health Worker (F)/ANM | 1 |
| 5. | Block Extension Educator | 1 |
| 6. | Health Assistant (M) | 1 |
| 7. | Health Assistant (F)/LHV | 1 |

*Contd...*

*Contd...*

| | | |
|---|---|---|
| 8. | LDC | 1 |
| 9. | Laboratory Technician | 1 |
| 10. | UDC | 1 |
| 11. | Driver | 1 |
| 12. | Class IV | 4 |
| | TOTAL | 15 |

## SUBCENTER

| Sl. No. | Post | Number |
|---|---|---|
| 1. | Health worker (female)/ANM | 1 |
| 2. | Health Worker (male) | 1 |
| 3. | Voluntary Worker | 1 |

# ASSIGNMENT–1 (A)
# ORIENTATION REPORT (URBAN)

Describe orientation report of urban community.

1. **Introduction.**

2. **Date of orientation.**

3. **Number of population.**

4. **Write down the definition and aims of community health center.**

5. **Write down the function of community health center.**

6. **Write down the definition and aims of primary health center.**

**7. Write down the function of primary health center.**

**8. Describe in detail of Anganwadi.**

- **Introduction of Anganwadi.**

- **Aims and objective of Anganwadi.**

**9. Write down the functions of Anganwadi.**

10. **Staffing pattern and time table schedule of Anganwadi.**

**Report.**

11. **Draw a diagram showing map of (urban) village.**

**(temples, private clinic, street, well, pond, school, pucca house [cemented], katcha house (noncemented), cinema, dairy, tower, market, shops, community health center [CHC], primary health center [PHC], subcenter [SC], anganwadi, panchayat, bank, etc.)**

## Diagram

# ASSIGNMENT–1 (B)
# ORIENTATION REPORT (URBAN)

Describe orientation report of urban community.

1. **Introduction.**

2. **Date of orientation.**

3. **Number of population.**

4. **Write down the definition and aims of community health center.**

5. **Write down the function of community health center.**

6. **Write down the definition and aims of primary health center.**

7. **Write down the function of primary health center.**

8. Describe in detail of Anganwadi.

- Introduction of Anganwadi.

- Aims and objective of Anganwadi.

9. Write down the functions of Anganwadi.

10. Staffing pattern and time table schedule of Anganwadi.

**Report**

11. **Draw a diagram showing map of (urban) village.**

    **(temples, private clinic, street, well, pond, school, pucca house [cemented], katcha house [noncemented], cinema, dairy, tower, market, shops, community health center [CHC], primary health center (PHC), subcenter [SC], anganwadi, panchayat, etc.)**

## Diagram

# ASSIGNMENT–1 (C)
# ORIENTATION REPORT (URBAN)

Describe orientation report of urban community.

1. **Introduction.**

2. **Date of orientation.**

3. **Number of population.**

4. **Write down the definition and aims of community health center.**

5. **Write down the function of community health center.**

6. **Write down the definition and aims of primary health center.**

7. **Write down the function of primary health center.**

8. **Describe in detail of Anganwadi.**

- **Introduction of Anganwadi**

- **Aims and objective of Anganwadi**

9. **Write down the functions of Anganwadi.**

10. **Staffing pattern and time table schedule of Anganwadi.**

**Report**

11. **Draw a diagram showing map of (urban) village.**

    **(temples, private clinic, street, well, pond, school, pucca house [cemented], katcha house [noncemented], cinema, dairy, tower, market, shops, community health center [CHC], primary health center [PHC], subcenter (SC), anganwadi, panchayat, etc.)**

## Diagram

# ASSIGNMENT–2 (A)
# ORIENTATION REPORT (RURAL)

Describe orientation report of rural community.

1. **Introduction.**

2. **Date of orientation.**

3. **Number of population.**

4. **Write down the definition and aims of community health center.**

5. **Write down the function of community health center.**

6. **Write down the definition and aims of primary health center.**

7. **Write down the function of primary health center.**

**8. Describe in detail of Anganwadi.**

**9. Write down the functions and staff of Anganwadi.**

**Report**

10. **Draw a diagram showing map of (urban) village.**

**(temples, private clinic, street, well, pond, school, pucca house [cemented], katcha house [noncemented], cinema, dairy, tower, market, shops, community health center [CHC], primary health center [PHC], subcenter [SC], anganwadi, panchayat, etc.)**

## Diagram

# ASSIGNMENT–2 (B)
# ORIENTATION REPORT (RURAL)

Describe orientation report of rural community.

1. **Introduction.**

2. **Date of orientation.**

3. **Number of population.**

4. **Write down the definition and aims of community health center.**

5. **Write down the function of community health center.**

6. **Write down the definition and aims of primary health center.**

7. **Write down the function of primary health center.**

**8. Describe in detail of Anganwadi.**

**9. Write down the functions and staff of Anganwadi.**

**Report**

10. **Draw a diagram showing map of (urban) village.**

    **(temples, private clinic, street, well, pond, school, pucca house [cemented], katcha house [noncemented], cinema, dairy, tower, market, shops, community health center [CHC], primary health center [PHC], subcenter [SC], anganwadi, panchayat, etc.)**

## Diagram

# ASSIGNMENT–2 (C)
# ORIENTATION REPORT (RURAL)

Describe orientation report of rural community.

1. **Introduction.**

2. **Date of orientation.**

3. **Number of population.**

4. **Write down the definition and aims of community health center.**

5. **Write down the function of community health center.**

6. **Write down the definition and aims of primary health center.**

7. **Write down the function of primary health center.**

8. **Describe in detail of Anganwadi.**

9. **Write down the functions and staff of Anganwadi.**

Report

10. **Draw a diagram showing map of (urban) village.**

    **(temples, private clinic, street, well, pond, school, pucca house [cemented], katcha house [noncemented], cinema, dairy, tower, market, shops, community health center [CHC], primary health center [PHC], subcenter [SC], anganwadi, panchayat, etc.)**

## Diagram

# ASSIGNMENT–3
## ORIENTATION REPORT (WATER PURIFICATION)

Visit to water supply and water purification.

1. **Introduction.**

2. **Date of orientation.**

3. **Place.**

4. **Purpose of visit.**

5. **Report.**

# ASSIGNMENT–4
# ORIENTATION REPORT (SEWAGE DISPOSAL)

Visit to sewage disposal

**1. Introduction.**

**2. Date of orientation.**

3. Place.

4. Purpose of visit.

5. Report.

# ASSIGNMENT–5
# ORIENTATION REPORT (MILK PLANTATION)

Visit to milk plantation

1. **Introduction.**

2. **Date of orientation.**

3. **Place.**

4. **Purpose of visit**

5. **Report**

# ASSIGNMENT–6
# ORIENTATION REPORT (SLAUGHTER HOUSE)

Visit to slaughter house

1. **Introduction.**

2. **Date of orientation.**

3. **Place.**

4. **Purpose of visit.**

5. **Report.**

# ASSIGNMENT–7
# ORIENTATION REPORT (COTTON MILLS)

Visit to cotton mill

1. **Introduction.**

2. **Date of orientation.**

3. Place.

4. Purpose of visit.

5. Report.

# ASSIGNMENT–8
# ORIENTATION REPORT (PHARMACY INDUSTRIES)

Visit to pharmacy industries

1. **Introduction.**

2. **Date of orientation.**

3. Place.

4. Purpose of visit.

5. Report.

## ASSIGNMENT–9
## ORIENTATION REPORT (WHEAT INDUSTRIES)

Visit to wheat industries

**1. Introduction.**

**2. Date of orientation.**

3. **Place.**

4. **Purpose of visit.**

**5. Report.**

# ASSIGNMENT–10
# ORIENTATION REPORT (SHOES INDUSTRIES)

Visit to shoes industries

1. **Introduction.**

2. **Date of orientation.**

3. **Place.**

**4. Purpose of visit.**

**5. Report.**

# ASSIGNMENT–11
# ORIENTATION REPORT (STEEL INDUSTRIES)

Visit to steel industries

**1. Introduction.**

**2. Date of orientation.**

3. **Place.**

4. **Purpose of visit.**

5. **Report.**

# 2. SURVEY OF RURAL AND URBAN COMMUNITY

Survey research is that which examines the characteristics, behavior, attitude and intention of a group of people by asking individuals belonging to that group (typically only a subject) to answer a series of questions.

Survey is descriptive and exploratory in nature. In that survey, information can be obtained from a large population in a fairly economical manner.

## TYPE OF SURVEY

- **Descriptive survey:** It is carried out for the purpose or subjects with specific characteristics. Descriptive studies usually entail the precise measurement of phenomena as they currently exist within a single group.
- **Exploratory survey:** The word 'explore' implies scrutinizing unknown regions for the purpose of discovery. Indeed exploratory studies serve this purpose and are particularly useful during the early stage of investigating the relationship between phenomena about which not much is known.
- **Explanatory survey:** These are conducted to provide causal explanation or phenomena or situations. According to Warwick and Lininger, the following three conditions must be satisfied to establish a causal explanation:
  1. The cause and effect must be associated with each other.
  2. The cause must proceed with effect.
  3. The other possible explanation of the effect should be ruled out.
- **Comparative survey:** Studies utilize set criteria to contrast two or more groups of designated variables. This popular type of survey has often been used by investigators to compare two distinct groups on the basis of such qualities of knowledge level, perceptions, or attitudes.
- **Evaluative survey:** This is also a descriptive, but it has the additional dimension of one or more criteria by which some evaluative judgment will be made about the respondents either individually or as groups.
- **Correlation survey:** This survey collects data on more than one variable from one group of respondents with the intent of estimating the magnitude of the relationships between the variables.

## PANCHAYATI RAJ INSTITUTIONS

The Panchayati Raj is a 3-tier structure of rural self-government in India, linking the village to the district. The three institutions are:

- Panchayat—at the village level
- Panchayat samiti—at the block level
- Zila parishad—at the district level.

The panchayati Raj institutions are accepted as agencies of public welfare. All development programs are channeled through these bodies.

### At the Village Level

The Panchayati Raj at the village level consists of:
- The gram sabha
- The gram panchayat
- The nyaya panchayat.
- **Gram Sabha:** It is the assembly of all adults of the village, which meets at least twice a year. The Gram Sabha considers proposals for taxation, discusses the annual program and elects members of the Gram Panchayat.
- **Gram Panchayat:** It is the executive organ of the Gram Sabha and an agency for planning and development at the village level. Its strength varies from 15 to 30 and the population covered also varies from 5,000 to 15,000 or more. The members of the panchayat hold office for a period of 3 to 4 years. Every panchayat has an elected president, a vice-president and a Panchayat Secretary. The powers and functions of the Panchayat Secretary are very wide—they cover the entire field of civic administration including sanitation, public health and of social and economic development of the village.
- **Nyaya Panchayat:** It is comprised of 5 members from the panchayat. It tries to solve dispute between two parties/groups/individuals over certain matters in mutual consent. Thus saves the troubles of going to formal judicial system.

### At the Block Level

A block consists of about 100 villages and a population of about 80,000 to 1,20,000. The Panchayat Raj agency at the block level is the panchayat samiti/janapada panchayat. The Panchayat Samiti consists of all Sarpanchas of the village panchayat at the block; MLAs, MPs residing in the block area; representatives of the women, scheduled caste, scheduled tribes and cooperative societies. The block development officer is the ex-officio secretary of the Panchayat Samiti. The prime function of the panchayat samiti is the execution of the community development program in the block level. The funds provided by the government for stage 1 and stage 2 developments are channeled through Panchayat Samiti. The block development officer and his staff give technical assistance and guidance to the village panchayat engaged in the development work.

### At the District Level

The Zila Parishad/Zila panchayat is the agency of rural local self-government at the district level. The members of the Zila Parishad include all heads of the panchayat samitis in the district; MPs, MLAs of the district, representatives of scheduled castes, scheduled tribes and women and 2 persons of experience in administration, public health or rural development. The Collector of the District is the non-voting member. Thus, the membership of Zila Parishad is fairly large varying from 40 to 70.

The Zila Parishad is primarily supervisory and coordinating body. Its function and powers vary from state to state. In some states, Zila Parishad is vested with administrative functions. Family Planning and MCH officers are under the control of the Zila Parishad.

## INDICATORS

### Introduction

Indicators are required to measure the health status of the community and to compare the health status of one country with that of another; for assessment of health care needs; for allocation of scarce resources and for monitoring and evaluation of health services activities and programs. Indicators help to measure the extent to which the objectives and targets of a program are being attained.

### Definition

Indicators are defined as variables, which help to measure changes.

### Characteristics of Indicators

- **Valid:** They should actually measure what they are supposing to measure.
- **Realiable:** The answers should be the same if measured different people in similar circumstances.

- **Sensitive:** They should be sensitive to changes in the situation concerned.
- **Feasible:** They should have the ability to obtain data needed.
- **Relevant:** They should contribute to the understanding of the phenomenon of interest.

## CLASSIFICATION OF HEALTH INDICATORS

### Mortality Indicators

- **Crude death rate:** The number of deaths per 1,000 population per year in given community.
- **Expectation of life:** The average number of years that will be lived by those born alive into a population, if the current age-specific mortality rate persists.
- **Infant mortality rate:** It is the ratio of deaths under 1year of age in a given year to the total number of live births in the same year; usually expressed as a rate per 1,000 live births.
- **Child mortality rate:** The number of deaths at ages 1 to 4 years in a given year, per 1,000 children in that age groups at the mid-point of the year concerned.
- **Under-5 proportionate mortality rate:** It is the proportion of total deaths occurring in the under-5 age group.
- **Maternal (puerperal) mortality rate:** The proportion of deaths among women of reproductive age.
- **Disease-specific mortality:** The mortality rates can be computed for specific diseases.
- **Proportional mortality rate:** The simplest measures estimating the burden of a disease in the community is proportional mortality rate, i.e. the proportion of all deaths currently attributed to it.

### Morbidity Indicators

- Incidence and prevalence
- Notification rates
- Attendance rates at out-patient departments, health centers, etc.
- Admission, readmission and discharge rates
- Duration of stay in hospital
- Spells of sickness or absence from work or school
- Disability rates
- Event-type indicators
- Number of days of restricted activity
- Bed disability days
- Work-loss days (or school loss days) within a specified period
- Person type indicators
- Limitation of mobility
- Limitation of activity.

### Nutritional Status Indicators

- Anthropometric measurements of preschool children
- Heights at school entry
- Prevalence of low birth weight (less than 2.5 kg).

### Health Care Delivery Indicators

- Proportion of GNP spent on health services
- Proportion of GNP spent on health-related activities
- Proportion of total health resources devoted to primary health care.

### Indicators of Quality of Life

Quality of life is difficult to define and even more difficult to measure. Various attempts have been made to reach one composite index from a number of health indicators. The physical quality of life index is one such index. It consolidates three indicators, viz. infant mortality, life expectancy at age one and literacy.

## Other Indicators Series

- Social indicators: It is divided into 12 categories.
  - Population
  - Family formation, families and households
  - Learning and educational services
  - Earning activities
  - Distribution of income, consumption and accumulation
  - Social security and welfare services
  - Health services and nutrition
  - Housing and its environment
  - Public order and safety
  - Time use; leisure and culture
  - Social stratification
  - Mobility.
- Basic need indicators
- Calorie consumption
- Access to water
- Life expectancy
- Death due to diseases
- Illiteracy
- Doctors and nurses per population
- Rooms per persons
- GNP per capita.
- Health for all indicators.

### *Health policy indicators*

- Political commitment to Health for All
- Resource allocation
- The degree of equity of distribution of health services
- Community involvement
- Organizational framework and managerial process

**Social and economical indicators related to health:**
- Rate of population increase
- GNP or GDP
- Income distribution
- Work condition
- Adult literacy rate
- Housing
- Food availability.

**Indicators for the provision of health care:**
- Availability
- Accessibility
- Utilization
- Quality of care.

**Health status indicators:**
- Low birth weight (percentage)
- Nutritional status and psychosocial development of children
- Infant mortality rate
- Child mortality rate (1–4 years)

- Life expectancy at birth
- Maternal mortality rate
- Disease specific mortality
- Morbidity incidence and prevalence
- Disability prevalence
- Millennium Development Goal Indicators.

The Millennium Development Goal adopted by the United Nations in the year 2000 provides an opportunity for concerted action to improve global health.

## CONCLUSION

There is no single comprehensive indicator of nation's health. Each available indicator reflects an aspect of health. The ideal index, which combines the effect of a number of components measured independently is yet to be developed.

# ASSIGNMENT–12 (A) SURVEY REPORT (URBAN/RURAL)

Describe survey report of rural/village community.

1. **Introduction.**

2. **Name of the village.**

3. **Date of visit.**

**4. Number of houses.**

**5. Total number of population.**

**6. Main occupation:** **Male**
**Female**

**7. Total number of males in village.**

**8. Total number of females in village.**

9. **Total number of old age:** **Male**
**Female**

10. **Total number of under-five age children:** **Newborn**
**Infant**
**Toddler**
**Adolescent**
**Preschool**

11. **Immunization.**

12. **Number of married:** **Male**
**Female**

13. **Number of eligible couples.**

14. **Total number of temporary family planning:** **Male**
**Female**

15. **Total number of permanent family planning:** **Male**
**Female**

16. Name of the hospital for delivery.

17. Type of house.

18. Type of water supply.

19. Educational status.

20. Spending leisure time.

21. **Electricity facility.**

22. **Disposal.**

23. **Number of antenatal mothers.**

24. **Number of postnatal mothers.**

25. **List of the communicable diseases in the community.**

## Describe about the gram sabha, gram panchayat and nyaya panchayat in the village.

1. **Gram sabha.**

2. **Gram panchayat.**

3. **Nyaya panchayat.**

4. **Mention the classification of health indicators in the village.**

## ASSIGNMENT–12 (B): SURVEY REPORT (RURAL)

Describe survey report of village community.

1. **Introduction.**

2. **Name of the village.**

3. **Date of visit.**

4. Number of houses.

5. Total number of population.

6. Main occupation: Male
Female

7. Total number of males in village.

8. Total number of females in village.

9. Total number of old age: Male
Female

10. Total number of under-five age children: Newborn
Infant
Toddler
Adolescent
Preschool

**11. Immunization.**

**12. Number of married:** **Male**
**Female**

**13. Number of eligible couples.**

**14. Total number of temporary family planning:** **Male**
**Female**

**15. Total number of permanent family planning:** **Male**
**Female**

**16. Name of the hospital for delivery.**

**17. Type of house.**

**18. Type of water supply.**

**19. Educational status.**

**20. Spending leisure time.**

**21. Electricity facility.**

**22. Disposal.**

**23. Number of antenatal mothers.**

**24. Number of postnatal mothers.**

**25. List of the communicable diseases in the community.**

## Describe about the gram sabha, gram panchayat and nyaya panchayat in the village.

**1. Gram sabha.**

**2. Gram panchayat.**

3. **Nyaya panchayat.**

4. **Mention the classification of health indicators in the village.**

## ASSIGNMENT–12 (C): SURVEY REPORT (RURAL)

Describe survey report of village community.

1. **Introduction.**

2. **Name of the village.**

3. **Date of visit.**

4. **Number of houses.**

5. **Total number of population.**

6. **Main occupation:** **Male**
**Female**

7. **Total number of males in village.**

8. **Total number of females in village.**

9. **Total number of old age:** **Male**
**Female**

10. **Total number of under-five age children:** **Newborn**
**Infant**
**Toddler**
**Adolescent**
**Preschool**

11. **Immunization.**

**12. Number of married:** **Male**
**Female**

**13. Number of eligible couples.**

**14. Total number of temporary family planning:** **Male**
**Female**

**15. Total number of permanent family planning:** **Male**
**Female**

**16. Name of the hospital for delivery.**

**17. Type of house.**

**18. Type of water supply.**

**19. Educational status.**

**20. Spending leisure time.**

**21. Electricity facility.**

**22. Disposal.**

**23. Number of antenatal mothers.**

**24. Number of postnatal mothers.**

**25. List of the communicable diseases in the community.**

Describe about the gram sabha, gram panchayat and nyaya panchayat in the village.

**1. Gram sabha.**

**2. Gram panchayat.**

**3. Nyaya panchayat.**

**4. Mention the classification of health indicators in the village.**

## ASSIGNMENT–12 (D): SURVEY REPORT (RURAL)

Describe survey report of village community.

1. **Introduction.**

2. **Name of the village.**

3. **Date of visit.**

4. **Number of houses.**

**5. Total number of population.**

**6. Main occupation:** **Male**
**Female**

**7. Total number of males in village.**

**8. Total number of females in village.**

**9. Total number of old age:** **Male**
**Female**

**10. Total number of under-five age children:** **Newborn**
**Infant**
**Toddler**
**Adolescent**
**Preschool**

**11. Immunization.**

12. **Number of married:** **Male**
**Female**

13. **Number of eligible couples.**

14. **Total number of temporary family planning:** **Male**
**Female**

15. **Total number of permanent family planning:** **Male**
**Female**

16. **Name of the hospital for delivery.**

17. **Type of house.**

18. Type of water supply.

19. Educational status.

20. Spending leisure time.

21. Electricity facility.

22. Disposal.

23. Number of antenatal mothers.

24. Number of postnatal mothers.

25. **List of the communicable diseases in the community.**

Describe about the gram sabha, gram panchayat and nyaya panchayat in the village.

1. **Gram sabha.**

2. **Gram panchayat.**

3. **Nyaya panchayat.**

4. **Mention the classification of health indicators in the village.**

## ASSIGNMENT–12 (E): SURVEY REPORT (RURAL)

Describe survey report of village community.

1. **Introduction.**

2. **Name of the village.**

3. **Date of visit.**

4. **Number of houses.**

**5. Total number of population.**

**6. Main occupation:** **Male**

**Female**

**7. Total number of males in village.**

**8. Total number of females in village.**

**9. Total number of old age:** **Male**

**Female**

**10. Total number of under-five age children:** **Newborn**
**Infant**
**Toddler**
**Adolescent**
**Preschool**

**11. Immunization.**

**12. Number of married:** **Male**
**Female**

**13. Number of eligible couples.**

**14. Total number of temporary family planning:** **Male**
**Female**

**15. Total number of permanent family planning:** **Male**
**Female**

**16. Name of the hospital for delivery.**

**17. Type of house.**

**18. Type of water supply.**

**19. Educational status.**

**20. Spending leisure time.**

**21. Electricity facility.**

**22. Disposal.**

**23. Number of antenatal mothers.**

**24. Number of postnatal mothers.**

**25. List of the communicable diseases in the community.**

## Describe about the gram sabha, gram panchayat and nyaya panchayat in the village.

**1. Gram sabha.**

**2. Gram panchayat.**

**3. Nyaya panchayat.**

**4. Mention the classification of health indicators in the village.**

## ASSIGNMENT–13 (A): SURVEY REPORT (URBAN)

Describe survey report of urban community.

1. **Introduction.**

2. **Name of the community.**

3. **Date of visit.**

4. **Number of houses.**

5. Total number of population.

6. Main occupation: Male
Female

7. Total number of males in community.

8. Total number of females in community.

9. Total number of old age: Male
Female

10. Total number of under-five age children: Newborn
Infant
Toddler
Adolescent
Preschool

11. Immunization.

**12. Number of married:** **Male**
**Female**

**13. Number of eligible couples.**

**14. Total number of temporary family planning:** **Male**
**Female**

**15. Total number of permanent family planning:** **Male**
**Female**

**16. Name of the hospitals for delivery.**

**17. Type of house.**

**18. Type of water supply.**

**19. Educational status.**

**20. Spending leisure time.**

**21. Electricity facility.**

**22. Disposal.**

**23. Number of antenatal mothers.**

**24. Number of postnatal mothers.**

25. **List of the communicable diseases in the community.**

## Describe about the gram sabha/zilla parishad, gram panchayat/nagar palika and nyaya panchayat/palika in the community.

1. **Gram sabha/zilla parishad.**

2. **Gram panchayat/nagar palika.**

3. **Nyaya panchayat/palika.**

**4. Mention the classification of health indicators in the community.**

## ASSIGNMENT–13 (B): SURVEY REPORT (URBAN)

Describe survey report of urban community.

1. **Introduction.**

2. **Name of the community.**

3. **Date of visit.**

4. **Number of houses.**

5. **Total number of population.**

6. **Main occupation:** **Male**
**Female**

7. **Total number of males in community.**

8. **Total number of females in community.**

9. **Total number of old age:** **Male**
**Female**

10. **Total number of under-five age children:** **Newborn**
**Infant**
**Toddler**
**Adolescent**
**Preschool**

11. **Immunization.**

**12. Number of married:** Male
Female

**13. Number of eligible couples.**

**14. Total number of temporary family planning:** Male
Female

**15. Total number of permanent family planning:** Male
Female

**16. Name of the hospital for delivery.**

**17. Type of house.**

18. Type of water supply.

19. Educational status.

20. Spending leisure time.

21. Electricity facility.

22. Disposal.

23. Number of antenatal mothers.

**24. Number of postnatal mothers.**

**25. List of the communicable disease in the community.**

Describe about the gram sabha/zilla parishad, gram panchayat/nagar palika and nyaya panchayat/palika in the community.

1. **Gram Sabha/Zilla Parishad.**

2. **Gram Panchayat/Nagar Palika.**

3. **Nyaya Panchayat/Palika.**

4. **Mention the classification of health indicators in the community.**

## ASSIGNMENT–13 (C): SURVEY REPORT (URBAN)

Describe survey report of urban community.

**1. Introduction.**

**2. Name of the community.**

**3. Date of visit.**

**4. Number of houses.**

**5. Total number of population.**

**6. Main occupation:** **Male**
**Female**

**7. Total number of males in community.**

**8. Total number of females in community.**

**9. Total number of old age:** **Male**
**Female**

**10. Total number of under-five age children:** **Newborn**
**Infant**
**Toddler**
**Adolescent**
**Preschool**

**11. Immunization.**

**12. Number of married:** **Male**
**Female**

**13. Number of eligible couples.**

14. **Total number of temporary family planning:** **Male**
**Female**

15. **Total number of permanent family planning:** **Male**
**Female**

16. **Name of the hospital for delivery.**

17. **Type of house.**

18. **Type of water supply.**

19. **Educational status.**

20. **Spending leisure time.**

21. **Electricity facility.**

22. **Disposal.**

23. **Number of antenatal mothers.**

24. **Number of postnatal mothers.**

25. **List of the communicable disease in the community.**

Describe about the gram sabha/zilla parishad, gram panchayat/nagar palika and nyaya panchayat/palika in the community.

1. **Gram Sabha/Zilla Parishad.**

2. **Gram Panchayat/Nagar Palika.**

3. **Nyaya Panchayat/Palika.**

4. **Mention the classification of health indicators in the community.**

## ASSIGNMENT–13 (D): SURVEY REPORT (URBAN)

Describe survey report of urban community.

1. **Introduction.**

2. **Name of the community.**

3. **Date of visit.**

4. **Number of houses.**

5. **Total number of population.**

6. **Main occupation:** **Male**
**Female**

7. **Total number of males in community.**

8. **Total number of females in community.**

9. **Total number of old age:** **Male**
**Female**

10. **Total number of under-five age children:** **Newborn**
**Infant**
**Toddler**
**Adolescent**
**Preschool**

11. **Immunization.**

**12. Number of married:** **Male**
**Female**

**13. Number of eligible couples.**

**14. Total number of temporary family planning:** **Male**
**Female**

**15. Total number of permanent family planning:** **Male**
**Female**

**16. Name of the hospital for delivery.**

**17. Type of house.**

**18. Type of water supply.**

**19. Educational status.**

**20. Spending leisure time.**

**21. Electricity facility.**

**22. Disposal.**

**23. Number of antenatal mothers.**

**24. Number of postnatal mothers.**

**25. List of the communicable disease in the community.**

## Describe about the gram sabha/zilla parishad, gram panchayat/nagar palika and nyaya panchayat/palika in the community.

**1. Gram Sabha/Zilla Parishad.**

**2. Gram Panchayat/Nagar Palika.**

**3. Nyaya Panchayat/Palika.**

**4. Mention the classification of health indicators in the community:**

## ASSIGNMENT–13 (E): SURVEY REPORT (URBAN)

Describe survey report of urban community.

1. **Introduction.**

2. **Name of the community.**

3. **Date of visit.**

4. **Number of houses.**

5. **Total number of population.**

6. **Main occupation:** **Male**
**Female**

7. **Total number of males in community.**

8. **Total number of females in community.**

9. **Total number of old age:** **Male**
**Female**

**10. Total number of under-five age children:** **Newborn**
**Infant**
**Toddler**
**Adolescent**
**Preschool**

**11. Immunization.**

**12. Number of married:** **Male**
**Female**

**13. Number of eligible couples.**

**14. Total number of temporary family planning:** **Male**
**Female**

**15. Total number of permanent family planning:** **Male**
**Female**

**16. Name of the hospital for delivery.**

**17. Type of house.**

18. **Type of water supply.**

19. **Educational status.**

20. **Spending leisure time.**

21. **Electricity facility.**

22. **Disposal.**

23. **Number of antenatal mothers.**

**24. Number of postnatal mothers.**

**25. List of the communicable disease in the community.**

Describe about the gram sabha, gram panchayat/nagar palika and nyaya panchayat/palika in the community.

1. **Gram Sabha/Zilla parishad.**

2. **Gram Panchayat/Nagar Palika.**

3. **Nyaya Panchayat/Palika.**

4. **Mention the classification of health indicators in the community.**

# 3. COMMUNITY HEALTH NURSING CONCEPT

## INTRODUCTION

Community health nursing is one of the professions, which operates within the realms of community health and helps in meeting health and nursing needs of the community. It plays a very important and challenging role in promoting and protecting health of people. Unlike other specialties of nursing, community health nursing lays major emphasis on primary level prevention and focuses on the entire community.

## DEFINITION

Community health nursing, a synthesis of both public health science and nursing science, is theoretically responsive to our prevailing ideas of social justice and the methods of distributing healthy care resources as chosen by the community (Archer Se 1982).

## PHILOSOPHY

1. **Philosophy of individual's right of being healty:** All humans having some nationally and internationally rights. The health care delivery system provides care to the people according to his/her rights.
2. **Philosophy of working together under a competent leader for the common good:** From child to adult, period, we are living together and fulfil the need, and in community health it is important to work together and understand needs of other people and fulfil their needs.
3. **Philosophy that people in the community have potential for continued development and are capable of dealing with their own problems, if educated and helped:** Every individual having own intelligence can lurk and deal with his/her needs. So based on this philosophy given on health education to individuals, they are capable for self-care.
4. **Philosophy of socialism:** All individuals live in society and society provides facility for production, distribution, e.g. food, housing, material production, education, health, transportation, etc. so without society and community individuals will not survive properly. Society and political system are responsible to plan and organize a system to provide services to all.

## OBJECTIVES

1. **To increase capability of community and to deal with their own health problems:** Increased by imparting adequate and desirable information and well-planned health education services for community at large and specific community groups on various health problems, health issues and topics.
2. **To strengthen community:** Resources—community resources include manpower, money, material, their development, distribution and utilization. Lack of resources, imbalanced distribution and improper utilization of resources have diverse impact on community health.
3. **To control and counteract environment:** This includes environment protection measures and changing reaction to environment when some protection measures are not feasible.

4. **To prevent and control communicable and non-communicable diseases:** This includes application of three levels of preventive measures for various health problems. These are primary level, secondary level and tertiary level measures.
5. **To provide specialized services:** To provide specialized services for mothers, children, adults, workers, elderly, handicapped and eligible couples.
6. **To conduct research:** To conduct research to build-up knowledge and contribute to further refinement and improvement of community health practice.
7. **To prepare** community for community health care services.

## PRINCIPLES

**Community health nursing is community focused, it is therefore essential to know the defined community, make a map and establish effective working relationship:** Community area; boundaries, important landmarks, people in general, community leaders, lifestyle, their resources, because this is important to easily assessment, so for this, map is very important to show the various places, which are present into community.

Community health nursing is based on identifying community health nursing needs and function within total community health program. Community health nursing must know the community needs and know the health care delivery system, health policy, health goals and objectives, health care programs, role of health personnel in various programs.

Health education, guidance and supervision are integral part of community health nursing. Health education is very important, it helps to improve health knowledge and skills and also improves positive attitude. Health teaching should be simple, understandable, specific, scientifically correct and practical value. Health service should be realistic in terms of available resources. Always plan, then provide service to the people based on health needs, money, material, man power. The health worker is accountable to the authorized health authority and functions within the policies, general goals and objectives set by the health agencies. Community health nurses or other health workers are employee of the central, state cooperation, municipality, local board, private or voluntary health agencies. They must function with the officer in charge. Effective health worker irrespective of position or place of work, functions as a team member. Team work is very important for providing adequate care. Community health nurses cooperate with other health worker and do the work easily and to maintain good relationship with the dais, anganwadi workers, ANM, etc.

In community health, community is in focus and then the individual, which is the unit of all health care services. People's health is influenced by various factors such as biological, lifestyle, environmental and resources. Family, not alone, is because with family setting, people having less anxiety, so focus on community than individual.

Professional relationship and etiquette are essential in community health services. Professional relationship is maintained with block development officer, ayurvedic, unani, homeopathic dispensaries, panchayat, voluntary organization, doctors, dais, anganwadi workers.

Community involvement is integral part of community health nursing practice. If community health nurse wants to provide good care in community in this condition, community involvement is very necessary because resources are not available to every person, so community involvement is necessary, e.g. village pradhan, panchayat member, block development officers, leader, religious group, teachers, mothers, elderly men and women and other family members.

Individual and families participate fully in all decision making relating to attendant of work. All family members and all community members are responsible for their own health, so it is important to take serious concern for own health and all family members fully participate with community health nurse for restoring health.

Continuous service is effective service and community health nurse must provide continuous health service. Community health nurse provides continuous care and observation.

Well-developed system of records and reports is essential for community health service. Records and report are very important by this community health nurse to maintain data of the patient and evaluate patient's condition easily.

Periodic and continuous appraisal and evaluation of health situation and health services are basic to community health nurse; health needs and problems change time to time and person to person so, time to time periodic and continuous assessment is very necessary.

Health services should be available and accessible to all without any discrimination. Every individual has a right to attain optimum health. Community health nurse should provide same care to all individuals without discrimination of color, caste and race.

Health worker should be non-political, non-sectorial in his and her relationship. Community health nurse should not be involved in politics and religion with differentiation, but she can respect all religions and understand all policies and not involved personally in all that.

Health worker must maintain professional dignity and must never accept any gift or bribe. Community health nurse must maintain professional relationship.

## GOALS AND FUNCTIONS OF COMMUNITY HEALTH NURSE

- Care provider
- Sensitive observer
- Educator
- Advocate
- Concern advisor
- Change agent
- Manager
- Planner
- Organizer
- Director and coordinator
- Controller and evaluator
- Leader
- Collaborator
- Researcher.

### Conceptual Framework

Conceptual framework/models are usually developed on the basis of either theories or assumptions and beliefs pertaining to the subject concerned.

Community health determinants.

- Human biology
- Lifestyle
- Environment
- Health resources
- Scope of community health nursing.

The scope of community health nursing that encompasses the goals and aims of community health services is the priority practice or service the focus of these priority practices and practice levels.

#### *The goals and aims*

- Promote and preserve health.
- Restore health.
- Improve quality life.

#### *The priority practices*

Community health programs are based on three classic levels of prevention (Level and Clark 1965). They are:

1. *Primary prevention:* Focuses on health promotion and prevention of disease or injury. Examples of primary prevention activities include child care clinic, immunization program, safety program, nutrition program.
2. *Secondary prevention:* Focuses on screening and early diagnosis of disease. Example of secondary intervention include tuberculosis and lead screening program.
3. *Tertiary prevention:* Focuses on optimizing function for children with disabilities or chronic diseases. Tertiary intervention includes rehabilitation and disease management program for asthma, sickle cell disease, cancer, anorexia, etc.

### *The focus on practice level*

Community health nursing, which is nursing aspect of organized community health practice, committed to goals of community health. It helps in achieving these goals by providing comprehensive health and nursing care services to the entire community. Thus community is the focus of the community health services.

## CONCEPT OF CONTROL

- Disease control
- The incidence of disease
- The duration of disease
- The effect of infection
- Financial burden in the community.

Control activity focuses a primary prevention or secondary prevention. Most control programs combine the two, i.e. concept of control or concept of prevention.

## PRINCIPLES OF EARLY DISEASE DETECTION

- The condition sought should be an important health problem
- There should be an accepted treatment for patient with recognized disease
- Facilities for diagnosis and treatment should be available
- There should be a recognizable latent or early symptomatic stage
- There should be a suitable test or examination
- The test should be acceptable to the population
- The natural history of the condition including development from latent to declared disease should be adequately understood
- There should be an agreed policy on whom to treat
- The cost of case finding should be economically balanced in relation to possible expenditures on medical care as a whole
- Case finding should be a continuing process and not a once and for all project.

# ASSIGNMENT–14 : PRIMARY PREVENTION

1. **What is primary prevention?**

2. **Discuss briefly strategies involved in primary prevention.**

3. **Discuss nursing intervention in primary prevention of communicable disease within the community.**

4. **Discuss nursing intervention in primary prevention of non-communicable disease within the community.**

# ASSIGNMENT–15 : SECONDARY PREVENTION

1. **What do you understand by secondary prevention?**

2. **Discuss briefly about secondary prevention.**

3. **Discuss nursing intervention in secondary prevention of communicable disease within the community.**

4. **Discuss nursing intervention in secondary prevention of non-communicable disease within the community.**

# ASSIGNMENT–16 : TERTIARY PREVENTION

1. **What is tertiary prevention?**

2. **What is disability limitation? Write down various types of rehabilitative aspects.**

3. **Define rehabilitation. Write down various types of rehabilitative aspects.**

4. **Discuss nursing role in tertiary prevention.**

# 4. COMMUNITY NURSING PROCESS

In community nursing, the focus of the nursing process shifts from the individual child and family to the community or target population. The stages of the process (assessment, diagnosis, planning, intervention, and evaluation) are similar, whether the client is a child or a population of children. Only the types of intervention and indication of wellness and illness differ (Anderson and McFarlane, 2000).

## COMMUNITY NEEDS ASSESSMENT

The assessment phase of the community nursing process is called community needs assessment. Assessment involves the collection of subjective and objective information about a community. Subjective information indicates what community members say are their most important needs and can be determined in a number of ways. One way is to distribute questionnaires to a sample of people living in the community, another way is to interview community member directly, phoning or meeting with individuals, such as community leaders, who represent the group or who have a special role in the group.

The nurse collects objective information or data either by direct observation or through written sources. A windshield tour is one method of direct observation. Nurses drive through a neighborhood and take notes about the environment, including the appearance of house, the presence of sidewalks and gutters, the number of public areas, etc.

## COMMUNITY DIAGNOSIS

A community health diagnosis is reflection of health status, risks or needs as determined by a causative agent. The format of community diagnosis is similar to an individual nursing diagnosis in that it identifies a problem (need) and the etiology related to that problem (causative agents ). An example of a community nursing diagnosis is 'child abuse related to a violent environment' (Visiting Nurses Association, 1986).

## COMMUNITY PLANNING

The nurse collaborates with community members in developing a plan that addresses the needs and problems of the target population. For example, a goal for preventing bicycle injuries is, 'within 1 year all students in the first grade will wear bicycle helmets.'

## COMMUNITY IMPLEMENTATION

During program implementation, the nurse and community members carry out the intervention. Whether the program is simple or complex, oversight is needed to ensure that everyone involved is communicating with each other, following the guideline of the plan, keeping within the timeline and documenting daily activities and expenses. The documenting will prove invaluable during the evaluation phases of the process.

## COMMUNITY EVALUATION

Evaluation identifies whether the goals and program objectives are met. Various models of program evaluation exist. A structure, process and outcome method is commonly used by health care organizations.

# ASSIGNMENT–17 (A): COMMUNITY NURSING PROCESS (RURAL)

Name: ________________ FF No: ________________

Age: ________________ Date of birth: ________________

1st year/2nd year/3rd year/4th year or ________________ years

Sex: ________________ Date of care started ________________

Head of the family: ________________ Date of care ended ________________

Address: ________________

| Assessment | Goal | Planning | Intervention | Evaluation |
|---|---|---|---|---|
| | | | | |

| Assessment | Goal | Planning | Intervention | Evaluation |
|---|---|---|---|---|
| | | | | |

| Assessment | Goal | Planning | Intervention | Evaluation |
|---|---|---|---|---|
| | | | | |

# ASSIGNMENT–17 (B): COMMUNITY NURSING PROCESS (URBAN)

Name: ______________________ FF No: ______________________

Age: ______________________ Date of birth: ______________________

1st year/2nd year/3rd year/4th year or ______________ years

Sex: ______________________ Date of care started: ______________________

Head of the family: ______________________ Date of care ended: ______________________

Address: ______________________________________________

| Assessment | Goal | Planning | Intervention | Evaluation |
|---|---|---|---|---|
| | | | | |

| Assessment | Goal | Planning | Intervention | Evaluation |
|---|---|---|---|---|
| | | | | |

| Assessment | Goal | Planning | Intervention | Evaluation |
|---|---|---|---|---|
| | | | | |

| Assessment | Goal | Planning | Intervention | Evaluation |
|---|---|---|---|---|
| | | | | |

# 5. HEALTH EDUCATION

## ASSIGNMENT–18 (A)

Deliver health education: ____________________

Topic: ____________________

Group: ____________________

Size of group: ____________________

Venue: ____________________

Date: ____________________

Time: ____________________

Previous knowledge: ____________________

Method of teaching: ____________________

AV aids: ____________________

General objectives: ____________________

| Time | Specific objectives | Content | Teaching and learning activities | AV aids | Evaluation |
|---|---|---|---|---|---|
| | | | | | |

| Time | Specific objectives | Content | Teaching and learning activities | AV aids | Evaluation |
|---|---|---|---|---|---|
| | | | | | |

| Time | Specific objectives | Content | Teaching and learning activities | AV aids | Evaluation |
|---|---|---|---|---|---|
| | | | | | |

| Time | Specific objectives | Content | Teaching and learning activities | AV aids | Evaluation |
|---|---|---|---|---|---|
| | | | | | |

# EVALUATION FOR HEALTH TALK

Name: ____________________

Audience: ____________________ Date: ____________________

No. of audience: ____________________ Time: ____________________

Topic: ____________________ Place: ____________________

Total marks: ____________________

| Sl. No. | Factors/Elements | 1 | 2 | 3 | 4 | 5 |
|---|---|---|---|---|---|---|
| 1. | The student's personal appearance | So-so | Improbable | Satisfactory | Good | Excellent |
| 2. | Poise | Seldom appeared | Some tension apparent | Yes/no | Most of the times | Always |
| 3. | Voice and clarity | Monotonous | Dull | Satisfactory | Pleasant | Lively |
| 4. | Distractive gestures/ mannerism | Almost/always | Usually | Sometimes | Not very often | Hardly ever |
| | **CONTENT AND PRESENTATION** | | | | | |
| 5. | Amount of material | Nothing worthwhile | Too much | Satisfactory | Well-planned | Very well planned and presented |
| 6. | Organization and explanation | Could not understand | Difficult to follow | Fairly clear | Clear | Very clear and easy to follow |
| 7. | Environment | Not considered important | Just thought of satisfactory | Organized | Well-organized | Very well-planned |
| 8. | Impressiveness | Practically nil | Occasionally just clear | Satisfactory, sometimes appropriate | Good | Very good |
| 9. | AV aids Blackboard | Too crowded illegible | Untidy, partly illegible | Satisfactory | Materials logically appropriate | Very well-maintained, appropriate |
| 10. | Diagram, charts and models | Not planned, not prepared | Just appropriate | Satisfactory | Appropriate | Very clear and informative |

**Teacher's sign**

## ASSIGNMENT–18 (B)

Deliver health education: __________

Topic: __________

Group: __________

Size of group: __________

Venue: __________

Date: __________

Time: __________

Previous knowledge: __________

Method of teaching: __________

AV aids: __________

General objectives: __________

| Time | Specific objectives | Content | Teaching and learning activities | AV aids | Evaluation |
|---|---|---|---|---|---|
| | | | | | |

| Time | Specific objectives | Content | Teaching and learning activities | AV aids | Evaluation |
|---|---|---|---|---|---|
| | | | | | |

| Time | Specific objectives | Content | Teaching and learning activities | AV aids | Evaluation |
|---|---|---|---|---|---|
| | | | | | |

| Time | Specific objectives | Content | Teaching and learning activities | AV aids | Evaluation |
|---|---|---|---|---|---|
| | | | | | |

| Time | Specific objectives | Content | Teaching and learning activities | AV aids | Evaluation |
|---|---|---|---|---|---|
| | | | | | |

# EVALUATION FOR HEALTH TALK

Name: ____________________

Audience: ____________________ Date: ____________________

No. of audience: ____________________ Time: ____________________

Topic: ____________________ Place: ____________________

Total marks: ____________________

| Sl. No. | Factors/elements | 1 | 2 | 3 | 4 | 5 |
|---|---|---|---|---|---|---|
| 1. | The student's personal appearance | So-so | Improbable | Satisfactory | Good | Excellent |
| 2. | Poise | Seldom appeared | Some tension apparent | Yes/No | Most of the times | Always |
| 3. | Voice and clarity | Monotonous | Dull | Satisfactory | Pleasant | Lively |
| 4. | Distractive gestures / mannerism | Almost/always | Usually | Sometimes | Not very often | Hardly ever |
| | **CONTENT AND PRESENTATION** | | | | | |
| 5. | Amount of material | Nothing worth-while | Too much | Satisfactory | Well-planned | Very well-planned and presented |
| 6. | Organization and explanation | Could not understand | Difficult to follow | Fairly clear | Clear | Very clear and easy to follow |
| 7. | Environment | Not considered important | Just thought of satisfactory | Organized | Well-organized | Very well-planned |
| 8. | Impressiveness | Practically nil | Occasionally just clear | Satisfactory, sometimes appropriate | Good | Very good |
| 9. | AV aids Blackboard | Too crowded illegible | Untidy, partly illegible | Satisfactory | Materials logically appropriate | Very well-maintained, appropriate |
| 10. | Diagram, charts and models | Not planned, not prepared | Just appropriate | Satisfactory | Appropriate | Very clear and informative |

**Teacher's sign**

## FAMILY FOLDER

I. Health Center : ____________________

Opened on Date : ____________________

Name of the Head of Family : ____________________

Closed on Date : ____________________

Religion/Caste : ____________________

Village : ____________________

1. Family Composition

House No : ____________________

a. Size of family : ____________________

address : ____________________

b. Joint/single : ____________________

____________________

## Family History

**Number of Family Members**

| Sl. No. | Name | Sex | Age | Relation to head of the family | Education | Occupation | Income Per month | Immunization status health status |
|---|---|---|---|---|---|---|---|---|
| | | | | | | | | |

II. Environment

1. **Housing**
   - Rented/own
   - No. of rooms
   - Persons per living room.
   - Dampness :Yes/No
   - Floor :Kutcha-Pucca other (specify)
   - Walls :Mud/Brick/With plaster/other (specify)
   - Roof :Thatched/Tiles/Sheets? Concrete/Other (specify)
   - Ventilation in living room: Good/Satisfactory/Poor
   - Kitchen :Separate/Not separate/Smoky/Smokeless
   - Cattle shed :Not required/None/Attached/Separate
   - Electricity :Yes/No Locality—Congested/Semi-congested/Open
2. **Drinking water source** – Well/Hand pump/Tube well/Other (specify)
3. **Excreta disposal** – Open field/Latrine/Other (specify)
4. **Refuse disposal** – Indiscriminate/Dumping/Composting/Other (specify)
5. **Insects and rodents:-**
   Files: Absent/present in large number/present in small number
   Mosquitoes: Absence/present in small number/present in large numbers
   Rodents: Absent/present in small number/present in large numbers
6. **Animals/pets owned**

III. Family Diet

| Diet consumed veg/non-veg/ mixed | Number of meals per day | Average/weekly/ration for whole family | | |
|---|---|---|---|---|
| Milk | ______ L | | | |
| Eggs | ________ g/kg | | | |
| Meat/Fish | _____ | | | |
| Rice | ________ g/kg | | | |
| Cereals, wheat, maize, bajra | ________ g/kg | | | |
| Sugar/jaggery | ____g/kg | | | |
| Fat/oils | ________ g/kg | | | |
| Vegetables | ________ g/kg | | | |
| Green leafy vegetables | ________ g/kg | | | |

## COMMENTS ON DIET

IV. Family Economics
- Number of earning members ______________________
- Dependency ration______________________
- Total family income per month Rs. ____________ per capita income per month ____________

**Per month expenditure on:**

(a) Food ______________________
(b) Housing ______________________
(c) Education ______________________
(d) Recreation ______________________
(e) Medical care ______________________
(f) Other ______________________

Total Rs. ______________________ per month
Saving ______________________

V. Social Problems
- Unemployment ______________________
- Indebtedness ______________________
- Unmarried ______________________
- Chronic sickness ______________________
- Old invalid dependants ______________________
- Other (specify) ______________________

VI. Utilization of Health Facility
- PHC ______________________
- Private practitioner ______________________
- Home remedies ______________________

VII. Field Notes (if any)

VII. Progress Report

(**Note:** Any improvement in the family in environment family dietary of any other characteristics)

| Date | Environment | Family dietary | Other | Signature |
|---|---|---|---|---|
| | | | | |

## FAMILY DATA COLLECTION CARD

Name of the Head of the House Hold : ____________________

Folder No. : ____________________

Address : ____________________

____________________

A copy of location of map of house : ____________________

**State your Aim and Objectives:**

**Date of 1st visit:**

- **Give a brief description of the family in terms of your observation.**

- **Describe the internal and external surroundings of the house, state the health risks and hazard identified, list your advice given to the family.**

- **State anticipated health needs, health related problems and your plan of actions.**

______________________________________________________________________
______________________________________________________________________
______________________________________________________________________
______________________________________________________________________
______________________________________________________________________
______________________________________________________________________
______________________________________________________________________
______________________________________________________________________
______________________________________________________________________
______________________________________________________________________

## I. Family Characteristics

1. Type of family : Nuclear/Joint/Extended
2. Size of family : ____________________
3. Religion : ____________________
4. State of origin : ____________________
5. Duration of stay (here) : ____________________
6. Monthly income (total) : ____________________
7. No of persons earning : ____________________
8. Source of income : ____________________
9. Monthly occupation : ____________________
10. Economic trade : ____________________
11. Status : ____________________
12. Chief diet : ____________________
13. Staple food : ____________________
14. Hobbies/leisure activities : ____________________
15. Psychosocial Reaction : ____________________

**Animals owned**

1 ____________ 2 ____________ 3 ____________

**Poultry owned**

1 ____________ 2 ____________ 3 ____________

**Pets owned**

1 ____________ 2 ____________

**Property owned**

1 ____________________
2 ____________________
3 ____________________
4 ____________________

**II. Housing Condition**

1. Types of house : Katcha/Pacca Own/Rented
2. No. of rooms : Presentence of varandah
3. Living space per head Presence of courtyard
4. Source of light : Condition of courtyard
5. Source of water :
6. Ventilation : Adequate/inadequate
7. Kitchen condition : Separate/Yes/No
8. Type : Chullah/Stove/Gas/Heater
9. Fuel used : Coal/Wood/Electricity/Oil
10. Storage of food :
11. Drainage system : Open/close
12. Disposal of water :
13. Domestic :
14. Human :
15. Domestic animal :
16. Shed : Inside/outside the house
17. Domestic pets : Yes/No specify :- Kitchen Garden, present/absent
18. Presence of trees : Yes/No specify
    shrubs : Yes/No

Measures for vector control ____________________

Vector nuisance : 1 ____________ 2 ____________

3 ____________ 4 ____________

Safe/unsafe For human health

Play facilities : Available indoor/outdoor

List accidents hazards : 1 ____________ 2 ____________

**III. Vital Events**

| During past 12 months | M | F |
|---|---|---|
| No. of births | | |
| No. of deaths | | |
| No. of abortions | | |
| No. of accidents | | |
| No. of pregnancies | | |
| No. of crimes/thefts | | |

**Causes of Disease/Death**

| Sl. No. | Age | Sex | Cause of episode | Health care |
|---|---|---|---|---|
| | | | | |
| | | | | |
| | | | | |
| | | | | |
| | | | | |
| | | | | |
| | | | | |
| | | | | |
| | | | | |
| | | | | |
| | | | | |
| | | | | |
| | | | | |
| | | | | |
| | | | | |
| | | | | |
| | | | | |
| | | | | |
| | | | | |
| | | | | |
| | | | | |
| | | | | |
| | | | | |
| | | | | |
| | | | | |
| | | | | |
| | | | | |
| | | | | |
| | | | | |
| | | | | |
| | | | | |

**Source of health care preferred** : ____________________

Military hospital : ____________________

Private practitioners : ____________________

Civil hospital : ____________________

Self care : ____________________

## GENERAL INFORMATION OF FAMILY MEMBERS
### (Persons living in the household)

| Sl. No. | Name | Relation with head of the family | Age | Sex | Marital | Status | Educational status | Occupation | Income | Present health status | Disability | Immunization | Health care taken | Remarks |
|---|---|---|---|---|---|---|---|---|---|---|---|---|---|---|
| | | | | | | | | | | | | | | |

**General Description of the members of the family not living in the household:**

A. Eligible couples identified in the family:

B. Eligible couple practices Family Planning Yes No

C. If Yes, specify

D. If No, state reason

**Roles of Family Members:**

**Q. What are the assigned household tasks?**

a. Adults

Male:

Female:

b. Children

Boy:

Girls:

______________________________________________

______________________________________________

______________________________________________

______________________________________________

______________________________________________

**Q. Relation of family members. How do they get along ?**

- Husband and wife ____________________
- Father and children ____________________
- Mother and children ____________________
- Children and children ____________________

**Q. Decision making in the family. Who makes the decision ?**

- Major decisions ____________________ (For e.g. hospitalization, family planning)
- Minor decision ____________________ (For e.g. errands to market, collection of rations).

## Comprehensive Family Health Care Study
## Antenatal and Postnatal Record

Name of the mother: ____________ Age: ____________ Religion: ____________

Husband's name: ____________ Age: ____________ Occupation: ____________

Address: ______________________________________________

______________________________________________

Gravida: ________ Para: ________ Date of LMP: ________ EDD: ________

### History of previous pregnancies

| No. | Age | Sex | FT/PM | Born alive/ Stillborn | Living/ dead | Healthy otherwise | Abortion in month | Pregnancy/ NA | Labor/NA | Puerperium/ NA |
|---|---|---|---|---|---|---|---|---|---|---|
| | | | | | | | | | | |

**Present pregnancy**

| Date | Height of uterus | Position presentation | Head fixed/ floating | FHR/m | Weight | Urine | | BP | Hb | Investigations |
|---|---|---|---|---|---|---|---|---|---|---|
| | | | | | | Albumin | Sugar | | | |
| | | | | | | | | | | Blood VDRL<br>Height<br>Nutrition<br>Heart<br>Lungs<br>Breasts<br>Abdomen<br>Anemia<br>Edema<br>Vaginal discharge<br>Other<br>Abnormalities |

| Date | Treatment | Health teaching | Remarks | Signature |
|---|---|---|---|---|
| | | | | |

## Internal

| Labor | Time | | | | |
|---|---|---|---|---|---|
| | Date | Hours | Minutes | | |
| Onset<br>Rupture of membranes<br>Birth of the child<br>Birth of placentas<br>Total hours<br>Nature of delivery | | | | | Membranes and placenta<br>Hemorrhage<br>Perineum-intact/lacerated<br>Episiotomy<br>Infant Sex<br>Wt Length<br>Head circumference<br>Condition at birth |

**Progress of the mother—postnatal**

| Date | Temp | Pulse | Resp | Height of uterus | Breasts | General condition and advice | Signature |
|---|---|---|---|---|---|---|---|
| | | | | | | | |

| Date | Progress of the child | Signature |
|---|---|---|
| | | |

# Comprehensive Family Health Care Study
## Infant and Child Health Record

Name: ____________________
Sex: ____________________
Age physical exam: ____________________

**If Normal, Mark 'O'; & If Abnormal, Mark 'X'**

- Father's name ____________________
- Mother's name ____________________
- Address ____________________
- Date of birth __________ Birth weight __________
- Birth history ____________________ normal/abnormal
- Birth attendant ____________________

| Month (Year) | Weight | Height | Month (Year) | Weight (kg) | Height (cm) |
|---|---|---|---|---|---|
| Jan | | | July | | |
| Feb | | | Aug | | |
| March | | | Sep | | |
| April | | | Oct | | |
| May | | | Nov | | |
| June | | | Dec | | |

## Immunizations

| Name of vaccine | Date | Date | Date | Date | Date |
|---|---|---|---|---|---|
| BCG | | | | | |
| DPT | | | | | |
| TAB | | | | | |
| Polio | | | | | |
| TT | | | | | |
| Cholera | | | | | |

## Development

| | Yes | No |
|---|---|---|
| Head raised | | |
| Rolls over | | |
| Eruption of tooth | | |
| Sat with support | | |
| Without support | | |
| Sat alone walked with support | | |
| Talked | | |
| Walked alone | | |
| Bladder control | | |
| Bowel control | | |

| Physical Exam | If Normal, Mark; 'O'; If Abnormal, Mark 'X' |
|---|---|
| Date<br>Age<br>Skin<br>Ears<br>Nose<br>Throat<br>Teeth and gum<br>Eyes<br>Bones<br>Joints<br>Liver<br>Spleen<br>Hb% | |
| **Dietary habits** | **Lab Investigation** |
| | |

**Signs of Malnutrition (if observed mark)**

- Xerosis
- Bitot's spot
- Keratomalacia
- Dermatitis

- Glossitis
- Angular stomatitis
- Bow legs
- Edema
- Others (specify)

## INFECTIOUS DISEASES

| | Age | Yes | No | Others (specify) | Age | Yes | No |
|---|---|---|---|---|---|---|---|
| - Primary Complex<br>- Chicken Pox<br>- Measles<br>- Whooping Cough<br>- Mumps | | | | | | | |

| Date | General Health: nutritional status, development and illness if any | Observation, treatment and health teaching | Sign of CH nurse |
|---|---|---|---|
| | | | |

## SCHOOL HEALTH SERVICE
### (Medical History Sheet)

Name of School: ______________________________

Name of Pupil: ______________________________

Standard: ______________________________

______________________________

______________________________

Age: Years: Sex: M/F:

Weight: ________ kg Hight: ________ cm Chest: ________ cm Expansion: ________ cm

General health and nutritional state: ______________________________

______________________________

Protective inoculations : TAB/vaccination

Physical defects/deformities: ______________________________

CVS: ______________________________

Respiratory system: ______________________________

GI system teeth: ______________________________

gums: ______________________________

liver: ______________________________

spleen: ______________________________

CNS: ______________________________

Eyes

Vision RE: ______________________________

LE: ______________________________

Ears RE: ______________________________

Hearing LE: ______________________________

Special Points: ______________________________

______________________________

______________________________

______________________________

______________________________

______________________________

______________________________

______________________________

______________________________

______________________________

______________________________

**Signature of Medical Officer/Principal**

## ADULTS HEALTH CARD

Name of head of family: ______________________________

House No: ______________________________

Village: ______________ Sex: ________ Year of Birth: ______________

Name: ______________________________

Marital status: ______________________________

Education: ______________________________

Occupation: ______________________________

______________________________

______________________________

Income: ______________________

| Immunizations date | Habits | Post illness |
|---|---|---|
| BCG ( )<br>TT ( )<br>TAB ( )<br>Cholera ( )<br>Others ( ) | Betel leaves ( )<br>Tobacco ( )<br>Smoking ( )<br>Alcohols ( )<br><br>Others (specify) ( ) | Vegetarian ( )<br>Tuberculosis ( )<br>STD ( )<br>Malaria ( )<br>Filaria ( )<br>Dysentery ( ) |

### Laboratory Investigations

| Date | Specimen Findings | Treatment | Signature |
|---|---|---|---|
| | | | |

## Morbidity

| Date | Complaints | Positive findings | Diagnosis | Treatment | Advice follow up | Signature |
|---|---|---|---|---|---|---|
| | | | | | | |

## Physical Health Assessment:

Height: __________ cm
Wt: ____________ kg
Resp. System:
CNS:
Per abdomen:
Bowels and bladder function:

General health and
Nutritional status

Eyes vision LE RE
Ears hearing LE RE
Temp. P R

Liver: ______________

Spleen: ______________

Muscle skeletal system:

Gait:

Mental and social health :
Adjustment aspects :
Family/Work :
General outlook :
Hobbies/interests :
Social circle :

Apparent physical/psychological defects
Special points:

# SECTION-2

BSc (N) Fourth (IV) Year,
Post Basic BSc (N), MSc (N)

# 6. COMMUNITY CASE STUDY

## ASSIGNMENT–19 (A)

Client's information: ____________________

Student information: ____________________

Name: ____________________

FF No. ____________________

Age: ____________ Date of birth: ____________

1st year/2nd year/3rd year/4th year ____________________

Sex: ____________ Date of care started: ____________

Head of the family: ____________ Date of care ended: ____________

Address: ____________________

**Introduction**
**General description**

**Family**

## Community Assessment

**Community setting**

1. Name of the area: Urban/rural
2. Name of the taluk/dist.
3. Population
4. Administration: Panchayat/Municipal
5. Main caste group
6. Occupation: Professional/non-professional skilled/agriculture
7. Method of recording births and deaths
8. Facilities available in the area and distance in kilometers
   a. Medical
      - Govt. Hospital
      - Private/Mission hospital
      - Private practitioners
   b. Social agencies
      - Red Cross, Lions Club, etc. and their activities in the area
9. Educational/run by whom—govt./private
10. Markets
11. Churches, temples, mosque
12. Recreation
13. Transportation: Roads, bus service
14. Library
15. Communication of health and/or development program, which are operating in the area
16. Influential persons in the area
17. Sanitation
    - Latrines (type—location, exereta disposal)
    - Waste water disposal
    - Refuse disposal
    - Disposal of the dead

## Family Assessment

**A. Home and family**

1. Family

| Name | Relationship to head of family | Age | Sex | Education | Occupation | Wages/salary | Health/status |
|---|---|---|---|---|---|---|---|
| | | | | | | | |

2. Property and income in addition to salary/wages
   a. Home: own/rented
      If rented amount
   b. Land: amount
      Land income
   c. Animal: kind
      Number
      Income
   d. Others (specify)
3. Family and social relationship:
   a. Attitudes among family members and neighbors
   b. Attitudes towards people of other community and religions
4. Description of house and surroundings
   a. Roof: Tiles/thatched/concrete
   b. Walls: Mud/brick/cement/other
   c. Floors: Mud/cement/other
   d. Number of rooms:
   e. Lighting: Oil lamps
   f. Furniture: Number/kind:
   g. Water supply: Well/tap/river/borewell
   h. Storage of food and water
   i. Washing place for vessels
   j. Bathing area—location and type

**B. Surroundings**

* Neatness and cleanliness
* Kitchen garden
* Trees and shrubs
* Where the animals are kept

**C. Health habits**

* Smoking
* Alcohol
* Drug, occasional, addiction

Family health attitudes, beliefs and practices with regard to:-

**I. Health problems (Disease):**

Cause and spread/type of medical aid sought/immunization/physical defects/others

______________________________________________

______________________________________________

______________________________________________

______________________________________________

______________________________________________

______________________________________________

______________________________________________

**II. Food problems:**

Hot/cold gas forming/others

______________________________________________

______________________________________________

______________________________________________

______________________________________________

______________________________________________

______________________________________________

______________________________________________

______________________________________________

**III. MCH problems:**

ANC/delivery/postpartum care/family care/newborn care/infant feeding

**IV. Vulnerable family members:**

**Nutritional assessment (24-hour recall)**

| Food items | Cooked amount | Raw amount | Calorie (kcal) | Protein (g) | Fat (g) | Calcium (mg) | Vitamin A (mg) | Iron (mg) |
|---|---|---|---|---|---|---|---|---|
| Breakfast<br>Midmorning<br>Lunch<br>Tea<br>Dinner | | | | | | | | |
| Total intake | | | | | | | | |
| Normal requirement | | | | | | | | |
| Deficit/excess | | | | | | | | |

$$\text{Degree of malnutrition} = \frac{\text{Actual weight of the child}}{\text{Expected weight}} \times 10$$

**Lab investigations**

| Sl. No. | Parameters | Normal value | In patients | Remark |
|---|---|---|---|---|
| | | | | |
| | | | | |
| | | | | |
| | | | | |
| | | | | |
| | | | | |
| | | | | |

**Family Care Plan Nursing process**

Name: ________________

Age: __________ sex: __________

| Health need | Nursing goals | Nursing intervention | Evaluation | Remarks of supervisor |
|---|---|---|---|---|
| | | | | |
| | | | | |
| | | | | |
| | | | | |
| | | | | |
| | | | | |
| | | | | |
| | | | | |
| | | | | |
| | | | | |
| | | | | |
| | | | | |
| | | | | |
| | | | | |
| | | | | |
| | | | | |
| | | | | |
| | | | | |
| | | | | |
| | | | | |
| | | | | |
| | | | | |
| | | | | |
| | | | | |
| | | | | |
| | | | | |
| | | | | |
| | | | | |
| | | | | |
| | | | | |
| | | | | |
| | | | | |
| | | | | |
| | | | | |

**Conclusion**

**Self-evaluation**

**Bibliography**

# ASSIGNMENT–19 (B): FAMILY CASE STUDY

Client's information: ______________________________

Student information: ______________________________

Name: ______________________________

FF No. ______________________________

Age: ____________ Date of birth: ____________

1st year/2nd year/3rd year/4th year ______________________________

Sex: ____________ Date of care started: ____________

Head of the family: ____________ Date of care ended: ____________

Address: ______________________________

______________________________

______________________________

**Introduction**

**General description**

______________________________

______________________________

______________________________

**Family**

______________________________

______________________________

______________________________

## Community Assessment

**Community setting**

1. Name of the area: Urban/rural
2. Name of the taluk/dist.
3. Population
4. Administration: Panchayat/Municipal
5. Main caste group
6. Occupation: Professional/non-professional skilled/agriculture
7. Method of recording births and deaths
8. Facilities available in the area and distance in kilometers
   a. Medical
      - Govt. Hospital
      - Private/Mission hospital
      - Private practitioners
   b. Social agencies
      - Red Cross, Lions Club, etc. and their activities in the area
9. Educational/run by whom—govt./private
10. Markets
11. Churches, temples, mosque

12. Recreation
13. Transportation: Roads, bus service
14. Library
15. Communication of health and/or development program, which are operating in the area
16. Influential persons in the area
17. Sanitation
    - Latrines (type—location, exereta disposal)
    - Waste water disposal
    - Refuse disposal
    - Disposal of the dead

## Family Assessment

**A. Home and family**

1. Family

| Name | Relationship to head of family | Age | Sex | Education | Occupation | Wages/salary | Health/status |
|---|---|---|---|---|---|---|---|
| | | | | | | | |

2. Property and income in addition to salary/wages
   a. Home: Own/rented
      If rented amount
   b. Land: Amount
      Land income
   c. Animal: Kind
      Number
      Income
   d. Others (specify)
3. Family and social relationship:
   a. Attitudes among family members and neighbors
   b. Attitudes towards people of other community and religions
4. Description of house and surroundings
   a. Roof: Tiles/thatched/concrete
   b. Walls: Mud/brick/cement/other
   c. Floors: Mud/cement/other
   d. Number of rooms:
   e. Lighting: Oil lamps
   f. Furniture: Number/kind
   g. Water supply: Well/tap/river/borewell
   h. Storage of food and water
   i. Washing place for vessels
   j. Bathing area—location and type

**B. Surroundings**
* Neatness and cleanliness
* Kitchen garden
* Trees and shrubs
* Where the animals are kept

Family health attitudes, beliefs and practices with regard to:

**C. Health habits**
* Smoking
* Alcohol
* Drug, occasional, addiction

**I. Health problems (Disease):**

Cause and spread/type of medical aid sought/immunization/physical defects/others

**II. Food problems:**

Hot/cold gas forming/others

**III. MCH problems:**

ANC/delivery/postpartum care/family care/newborn care/infant feeding

**IV. Vulnerable family members:**

Nutritional assessment (24 hours recall)

| Food Items | Cooked Amount | Raw Amount | Calorie (kcal) | Protein (g) | Fat (g) | Calcium (mg) | Vitamin A (mg) | Iron (mg) |
|---|---|---|---|---|---|---|---|---|
| Breakfast<br>Midmorning<br>Lunch<br>Tea<br>Dinner | | | | | | | | |
| Total intake | | | | | | | | |
| Normal requirement | | | | | | | | |
| Deficit/ excess | | | | | | | | |

$$\text{Degree of malnutrition} = \frac{\text{Actual weight of the child}}{\text{Expected weight}} \times 10$$

**Lab investigations**

| Sl. No. | Parameters | Normal value | In patients | Remark |
|---|---|---|---|---|
| | | | | |
| | | | | |
| | | | | |
| | | | | |
| | | | | |
| | | | | |
| | | | | |
| | | | | |
| | | | | |
| | | | | |
| | | | | |
| | | | | |
| | | | | |
| | | | | |
| | | | | |
| | | | | |
| | | | | |
| | | | | |
| | | | | |
| | | | | |
| | | | | |

**Family Care Plan Nursing process**

Name: ______________________________

Age: __________ Sex: __________

| Health need | Nursing goals | Nursing intervention | Evaluation | Remarks of supervisor |
|---|---|---|---|---|
| | | | | |
| | | | | |
| | | | | |
| | | | | |
| | | | | |
| | | | | |
| | | | | |
| | | | | |
| | | | | |
| | | | | |
| | | | | |
| | | | | |
| | | | | |
| | | | | |
| | | | | |
| | | | | |
| | | | | |
| | | | | |
| | | | | |
| | | | | |
| | | | | |
| | | | | |
| | | | | |
| | | | | |
| | | | | |
| | | | | |
| | | | | |
| | | | | |
| | | | | |
| | | | | |
| | | | | |
| | | | | |
| | | | | |
| | | | | |
| | | | | |

| Health need | Nursing goals | Nursing intervention | Evaluation | Remarks of supervisor |
|---|---|---|---|---|
| | | | | |
| | | | | |
| | | | | |
| | | | | |
| | | | | |
| | | | | |
| | | | | |
| | | | | |
| | | | | |
| | | | | |
| | | | | |
| | | | | |
| | | | | |
| | | | | |
| | | | | |
| | | | | |
| | | | | |
| | | | | |
| | | | | |
| | | | | |
| | | | | |
| | | | | |
| | | | | |
| | | | | |
| | | | | |
| | | | | |
| | | | | |
| | | | | |
| | | | | |
| | | | | |
| | | | | |
| | | | | |
| | | | | |
| | | | | |

| Health need | Nursing goals | Nursing intervention | Evaluation | Remarks of supervisor |
|---|---|---|---|---|
| | | | | |
| | | | | |
| | | | | |
| | | | | |
| | | | | |
| | | | | |
| | | | | |
| | | | | |
| | | | | |
| | | | | |
| | | | | |
| | | | | |
| | | | | |
| | | | | |
| | | | | |
| | | | | |
| | | | | |
| | | | | |
| | | | | |
| | | | | |
| | | | | |
| | | | | |
| | | | | |
| | | | | |
| | | | | |
| | | | | |
| | | | | |
| | | | | |
| | | | | |
| | | | | |
| | | | | |
| | | | | |
| | | | | |
| | | | | |

**Conclusion**

**Self-evaluation**

**Bibliography**

# ASSIGNMENT–19 (C): FAMILY CASE STUDY

Client's information: ____________________

Student information: ____________________

Name: ____________________

FFNo. ____________________

Age: ____________________ Date of birth: ____________________

1st year/2nd year/3rd year/4th year ____________________

Sex: ____________________ Date of care started: ____________________

Head of the family: ____________________ Date of care ended: ____________________

Address: ____________________

**Introduction**

**General description**

**Family**

## Community Assessment

**Community setting**

1. Name of the area: Urban/rural
2. Name of the taluk/dist.
3. Population
4. Administration: Panchayat/Municipal
5. Main caste group
6. Occupation: Professional/non-professional skilled/agriculture
7. Method of recording births and deaths
8. Facilities available in the area and distance in kilometers
   a. Medical
      - Govt. Hospital
      - Private/Mission hospital
      - Private practitioners
   b. Social agencies
      - Red Cross, Lions Club, etc. and their activities in the area
9. Educational/run by whom—govt./private
10. Markets
11. Churches, temples, mosque

12. Recreation
13. Transportation: Roads, bus service
14. Library
15. Communication of health and/or development program, which are operating in the area
16. Influential persons in the area
17. Sanitation
    - Latrines (type—location, exereta disposal)
    - Waste water disposal
    - Refuse disposal
    - Disposal of the dead

## Family Assessment

**A. Home and family**

1. Family

| Name | Relationship to head of family | Age | Sex | Education | Occupation | Wages/salary | Health/status |
|---|---|---|---|---|---|---|---|
| | | | | | | | |

2. Property and income in addition to salary/wages
    a. Home: Own/rented
    If rented, amount
    b. Land: Amount
    Land income
    c. Animal:
    Kind
    Number
    Income
    d. Others (specify)
3. Family and social relationship:
    a. Attitudes among family members and neighbors
    b. Attitudes towards people of other community and religions
4. Description of house and surroundings
    a. Roof: Tiles/thatched/concrete
    b. Walls: Mud/brick/cement/other
    c. Floors: Mud/cement/other
    d. Number of rooms:
    e. Lighting: Oil lamps
    f. Furniture: Number/kind:
    g. Water supply: Well/tap/river/borewell
    h. Storage of food and water

i. Washing place for vessels
j. Bathing area—location and type

**B. Surroundings:**
* Neatness and cleanliness
* Kitchen garden
* Trees and shrubs
* Where the animals are kept

**C. Health habits**
* Smoking
* Alcohol
* Drug, occasional, addiction

**Family health attitudes, beliefs and practices with regard to:**

**I. Health problems (Disease):**
Cause and spread/type of medical aid sought/immunization/physical defects/others

**II. Food problems:**
Hot/cold gas forming/others

**III. MCH problems:**
ANC/delivery/postpartum care/family care/newborn care/infant feeding

**IV. Vulnerable family members:**

**Nutritional assessment (24 hours recall)**

| Food Items | Cooked Amount | Raw Amount | Calorie (kcal) | Protein (g) | Fat (g) | Calcium (mg) | Vitamin A (mg) | Iron (mg) |
|---|---|---|---|---|---|---|---|---|
| Breakfast<br>Midmorning<br>Lunch<br>Tea<br>Dinner | | | | | | | | |
| Total intake | | | | | | | | |
| Normal requirement | | | | | | | | |
| Deficit/ excess | | | | | | | | |

$$\text{Degree of malnutrition} = \frac{\text{Actual weight of the child}}{\text{Expected weight}} \times 10$$

**Lab investigations**

| Sl. No. | Parameters | Normal value | Inpatients | Remark |
|---|---|---|---|---|
| | | | | |
| | | | | |
| | | | | |
| | | | | |
| | | | | |
| | | | | |
| | | | | |
| | | | | |
| | | | | |
| | | | | |
| | | | | |
| | | | | |
| | | | | |
| | | | | |
| | | | | |
| | | | | |
| | | | | |
| | | | | |
| | | | | |
| | | | | |
| | | | | |
| | | | | |

**Family Care Plan Nursing process**

Name: ____________________________________________

Age: ____________________ Sex: ______________________

| Health need | Nursing goals | Nursing intervention | Evaluation | Remarks of supervisor |
|---|---|---|---|---|
| | | | | |
| | | | | |
| | | | | |
| | | | | |
| | | | | |
| | | | | |
| | | | | |
| | | | | |
| | | | | |
| | | | | |
| | | | | |
| | | | | |
| | | | | |
| | | | | |
| | | | | |
| | | | | |
| | | | | |
| | | | | |
| | | | | |
| | | | | |
| | | | | |
| | | | | |
| | | | | |
| | | | | |
| | | | | |
| | | | | |
| | | | | |
| | | | | |
| | | | | |
| | | | | |
| | | | | |
| | | | | |
| | | | | |
| | | | | |
| | | | | |

| Health need | Nursing goals | Nursing intervention | Evaluation | Remarks of supervisor |
|---|---|---|---|---|
| | | | | |
| | | | | |
| | | | | |
| | | | | |
| | | | | |
| | | | | |
| | | | | |
| | | | | |
| | | | | |
| | | | | |
| | | | | |
| | | | | |
| | | | | |
| | | | | |
| | | | | |
| | | | | |
| | | | | |
| | | | | |
| | | | | |
| | | | | |
| | | | | |
| | | | | |
| | | | | |
| | | | | |
| | | | | |
| | | | | |
| | | | | |
| | | | | |
| | | | | |
| | | | | |
| | | | | |
| | | | | |
| | | | | |
| | | | | |
| | | | | |
| | | | | |
| | | | | |
| | | | | |
| | | | | |
| | | | | |

| Health need | Nursing goals | Nursing intervention | Evaluation | Remarks of supervisor |
|---|---|---|---|---|
| | | | | |
| | | | | |
| | | | | |
| | | | | |
| | | | | |
| | | | | |
| | | | | |
| | | | | |
| | | | | |
| | | | | |
| | | | | |
| | | | | |
| | | | | |
| | | | | |
| | | | | |
| | | | | |
| | | | | |
| | | | | |
| | | | | |
| | | | | |
| | | | | |
| | | | | |
| | | | | |
| | | | | |
| | | | | |
| | | | | |
| | | | | |
| | | | | |
| | | | | |
| | | | | |
| | | | | |
| | | | | |
| | | | | |
| | | | | |
| | | | | |
| | | | | |
| | | | | |
| | | | | |
| | | | | |
| | | | | |

**Conclusion**

**Self-evaluation**

**Bibliography**

## ASSIGNMENT–19 (D): FAMILY CASE STUDY

Client's information: ______________________________

Student information: ______________________________

Name: ______________________________

FFNo. ______________________________

Age: ______________ Date of birth: ______________

1st year/2nd year/3rd year/4th year ______________________________

Sex: ______________ Date of care started: ______________

Head of the family: ______________ Date of care ended: ______________

Address: ______________________________

**Introduction**

**General description**

**Family**

### Community Assessment

**Community setting**

1. Name of the area: Urban/rural
2. Name of the taluk/dist.
3. Population
4. Administration: Panchayat/Municipal
5. Main caste group
6. Occupation: Professional/non-professional skilled/agriculture
7. Method of recording births and deaths
8. Facilities available in the area and distance in kilometers
    a. Medical
        - Govt. Hospital
        - Private/Mission hospital
        - Private practitioners
    b. Social agencies
        - Red Cross, Lions Club, etc. and their activities in the area

9. Educational/run by whom—govt./private
10. Markets
11. Churches, temples, mosque
12. Recreation
13. Transportation: Roads, bus service
14. Library
15. Communication of health and/or development program, which are operating in the area
16. Influential persons in the area
17. Sanitation
    - Latrines (type—location, exereta disposal)
    - Waste water disposal
    - Refuse disposal
    - Disposal of the dead

## Family Assessment

**A. Home and family**

1. Family

| Name | Relationship to head of family | Age | Sex | Education | Occupation | Wages/salary | Health/status |
|---|---|---|---|---|---|---|---|
| | | | | | | | |

2. Property and income in addition to salary/wages
   a. Home: Own/rented
      If rented, amount
   b. Land: Amount
      Land income
   c. Animal:
      Kind
      Number
      Income
   d. Others (specify)
3. Family and social relationship:
   a. Attitudes among family members and neighbors
   b. Attitudes towards people of other community and religions
4. Description of house and surroundings
   a. Roof: Tiles/thatched/concrete
   b. Walls: Mud/brick/cement/other
   c. Floors: Mud/cement/other
   d. Number of rooms:
   e. Lighting: Oil lamps

f. Furniture: Number/kind:
g. Water supply: Well/tap/river/borewell
h. Storage of food and water
i. Washing place for vessels
j. Bathing area—location and type

**B. Surroundings**
* Neatness and cleanliness
* Kitchen garden
* Trees and shrubs
* Where the animals are kept

**C. Health habits**
* Smoking
* Alcohol
* Drug, occasional, addiction

**Family health attitudes, beliefs and practices with regard to:**

**I. Health problems (Disease):**

Cause and spread/type of medical aid sought/immunization/physical defects/others

**II. Food problems:**

Hot/cold gas forming/others

**III. MCH problems:**

ANC/delivery/postpartum care/family care/newborn care/infant feeding

**IV. Vulnerable family members:**

Nutritional assessment (24 hours recall)

| Food items | Cooked amount | Raw amount | Calorie (kcal) | Protein (g) | Fat (g) | Calcium (mg) | Vitamin A (mg) | Iron (mg) |
|---|---|---|---|---|---|---|---|---|
| Breakfast<br>Midmorning Lunch<br>Tea<br>Dinner | | | | | | | | |
| Total intake | | | | | | | | |
| Normal requirement | | | | | | | | |
| Deficit/ excess | | | | | | | | |

$$\text{Degree of malnutrition} = \frac{\text{Actual weight of the child}}{\text{Expected weight}} \times 10$$

**Lab investigations**

| Sl. No. | Parameters | Normal value | In patients | Remark |
|---|---|---|---|---|
| | | | | |
| | | | | |
| | | | | |
| | | | | |
| | | | | |
| | | | | |
| | | | | |
| | | | | |
| | | | | |
| | | | | |
| | | | | |
| | | | | |
| | | | | |
| | | | | |
| | | | | |
| | | | | |
| | | | | |
| | | | | |
| | | | | |
| | | | | |
| | | | | |

Family Care Plan Nursing process

Name: ____________________

Age: ____________ Sex: ____________

| Health need | Nursing goals | Nursing intervention | Evaluation | Remarks of supervisor |
|---|---|---|---|---|
| | | | | |

| Health need | Nursing goals | Nursing intervention | Evaluation | Remarks of supervisor |
|---|---|---|---|---|
| | | | | |
| | | | | |
| | | | | |
| | | | | |
| | | | | |
| | | | | |
| | | | | |
| | | | | |
| | | | | |
| | | | | |
| | | | | |
| | | | | |
| | | | | |
| | | | | |
| | | | | |
| | | | | |
| | | | | |
| | | | | |
| | | | | |
| | | | | |
| | | | | |
| | | | | |
| | | | | |
| | | | | |
| | | | | |
| | | | | |
| | | | | |
| | | | | |
| | | | | |
| | | | | |
| | | | | |
| | | | | |
| | | | | |
| | | | | |
| | | | | |
| | | | | |
| | | | | |

| Health need | Nursing goals | Nursing intervention | Evaluation | Remarks of supervisor |
|---|---|---|---|---|
| | | | | |
| | | | | |
| | | | | |
| | | | | |
| | | | | |
| | | | | |
| | | | | |
| | | | | |
| | | | | |
| | | | | |
| | | | | |
| | | | | |
| | | | | |
| | | | | |
| | | | | |
| | | | | |
| | | | | |
| | | | | |
| | | | | |
| | | | | |
| | | | | |
| | | | | |
| | | | | |
| | | | | |
| | | | | |
| | | | | |
| | | | | |
| | | | | |
| | | | | |
| | | | | |
| | | | | |
| | | | | |
| | | | | |
| | | | | |
| | | | | |
| | | | | |
| | | | | |

| Health need | Nursing goals | Nursing intervention | Evaluation | Remarks of supervisor |
|---|---|---|---|---|
| | | | | |
| | | | | |
| | | | | |
| | | | | |
| | | | | |
| | | | | |
| | | | | |
| | | | | |
| | | | | |
| | | | | |
| | | | | |
| | | | | |
| | | | | |
| | | | | |
| | | | | |
| | | | | |
| | | | | |
| | | | | |
| | | | | |
| | | | | |
| | | | | |
| | | | | |
| | | | | |
| | | | | |
| | | | | |
| | | | | |
| | | | | |
| | | | | |
| | | | | |
| | | | | |
| | | | | |
| | | | | |
| | | | | |
| | | | | |
| | | | | |
| | | | | |
| | | | | |

**Conclusion**

**Self-evaluation**

**Bibliography**

## ASSIGNMENT–19 (E): FAMILY CASE STUDY

Client's information: ______________________________

Student information: ______________________________

Name: ______________________________

FFNo. ______________________________

Age: ______________ Date of birth: ______________

1st year/2nd year/3rd year/4th year ______________________________

Sex: ______________ Date of care started: ______________

Head of the family: ______________ Date of care ended: ______________

Address: ______________________________

______________________________

______________________________

______________________________

### Introduction

General description

______________________________

______________________________

______________________________

______________________________

______________________________

### Family

______________________________

______________________________

______________________________

______________________________

______________________________

## Community Assessment

**Community setting**

1. Name of the area: Urban/rural
2. Name of the taluk/dist.
3. Population
4. Administration: Panchayat/Municipal
5. Main caste group
6. Occupation: Professional/non-professional skilled/agriculture
7. Method of recording births and deaths
8. Facilities available in the area and distance in kilometers
    a. Medical
        - Govt. Hospital
        - Private/Mission hospital
        - Private practitioners
    b. Social agencies
        - Red Cross, Lions Club, etc. and their activities in the area

9. Educational/run by whom—govt./private
10. Markets
11. Churches, temples, mosque
12. Recreation
13. Transportation: Roads, bus service
14. Library
15. Communication of health and/or development program, which are operating in the area
16. Influential persons in the area
17. Sanitation
    - Latrines (type—location, exereta disposal)
    - Waste water disposal
    - Refuse disposal
    - Disposal of the dead

## Family Assessment

**A. Home and family**

1. Family

| Name | Relationship to head of family | Age | Sex | Education | Occupation | Wages/salary | Health/status |
|---|---|---|---|---|---|---|---|
| | | | | | | | |

2. Property and income in addition to salary/wages
    a. Home: Own/rented
    If rented, amount
    b. Land: Amount
    Land income
    c. Animal:
    Kind
    Number
    Income
    d. Others (specify)
3. Family and social relationship:
    a. Attitudes among family members and neighbors
    b. Attitudes towards people of other community and religions
4. Description of house and surroundings
    a. Roof: Tiles/thatched/concrete
    b. Walls: Mud/brick/cement/other
    c. Floors: Mud/cement/other
    d. Number of rooms:

e. Lighting: Oil lamps
f. Furniture: Number/kind:
g. Water supply: Well/tap/river/borewell
h. Storage of food and water
i. Washing place for vessels
j. Bathing area—location and type

**B. Surroundings**

* Neatness and cleanliness
* Kitchen garden
* Trees and shrubs
* Where the animals are kept

**C. Health habits**

* Smoking
* Alcohol
* Drug, occasional, addiction

**Family health attitudes, beliefs and practices with regard to:-**

**I. Health problems (Disease):**

Cause and spread/type of medical aid sought/immunization/physical defects/others

**II. Food problems:**

Hot/cold gas forming/others

**III. MCH problems:**

ANC/delivery/postpartum care/family care/newborn care/infant feeding

**IV. Vulnerable family members:**

Nutritional assessment (24 hours recall)

| Food Items | Cooked amount | Raw amount | Calorie (kcal) | Protein (g) | Fat (g) | Calcium (mg) | Vitamin A (mg) | Iron (mg) |
|---|---|---|---|---|---|---|---|---|
| Breakfast<br>Midmorning<br>Lunch<br>Tea<br>Dinner | | | | | | | | |
| Total intake | | | | | | | | |
| Normal requirement | | | | | | | | |
| Deficit/excess | | | | | | | | |

$$\text{Degree of malnutrition} = \frac{\text{Actual weight of the child}}{\text{Expected weight}} \times 10$$

**Lab investigations**

| Sl. No. | Parameters | Normal value | Inpatients | Remark |
|---|---|---|---|---|
| | | | | |
| | | | | |
| | | | | |
| | | | | |
| | | | | |
| | | | | |
| | | | | |
| | | | | |
| | | | | |
| | | | | |
| | | | | |
| | | | | |
| | | | | |
| | | | | |
| | | | | |
| | | | | |
| | | | | |
| | | | | |
| | | | | |
| | | | | |
| | | | | |
| | | | | |
| | | | | |
| | | | | |

**Family Care Plan Nursing process**

Name: ______________________________

Age: ______________ Sex: ______________

| Health need | Nursing goals | Nursing intervention | Evaluation | Remarks of supervisor |
|---|---|---|---|---|
| | | | | |
| | | | | |
| | | | | |
| | | | | |
| | | | | |
| | | | | |
| | | | | |
| | | | | |
| | | | | |
| | | | | |
| | | | | |
| | | | | |
| | | | | |
| | | | | |
| | | | | |
| | | | | |
| | | | | |
| | | | | |
| | | | | |
| | | | | |
| | | | | |
| | | | | |
| | | | | |
| | | | | |
| | | | | |
| | | | | |
| | | | | |
| | | | | |
| | | | | |
| | | | | |
| | | | | |
| | | | | |
| | | | | |
| | | | | |

| Health need | Nursing goals | Nursing intervention | Evaluation | Remarks of supervisor |
|---|---|---|---|---|
| | | | | |
| | | | | |
| | | | | |
| | | | | |
| | | | | |
| | | | | |
| | | | | |
| | | | | |
| | | | | |
| | | | | |
| | | | | |
| | | | | |
| | | | | |
| | | | | |
| | | | | |
| | | | | |
| | | | | |
| | | | | |
| | | | | |
| | | | | |
| | | | | |
| | | | | |
| | | | | |
| | | | | |
| | | | | |
| | | | | |
| | | | | |
| | | | | |
| | | | | |
| | | | | |
| | | | | |
| | | | | |
| | | | | |
| | | | | |
| | | | | |
| | | | | |
| | | | | |

| Health need | Nursing goals | Nursing intervention | Evaluation | Remarks of supervisor |
|---|---|---|---|---|
| | | | | |
| | | | | |
| | | | | |
| | | | | |
| | | | | |
| | | | | |
| | | | | |
| | | | | |
| | | | | |
| | | | | |
| | | | | |
| | | | | |
| | | | | |
| | | | | |
| | | | | |
| | | | | |
| | | | | |
| | | | | |
| | | | | |
| | | | | |
| | | | | |
| | | | | |
| | | | | |
| | | | | |
| | | | | |
| | | | | |
| | | | | |
| | | | | |
| | | | | |
| | | | | |
| | | | | |
| | | | | |
| | | | | |
| | | | | |
| | | | | |
| | | | | |
| | | | | |

**Conclusion**

**Self-evaluation**

**Bibliography**

# 7. HEALTH ASSESSMENT

## INTRODUCTION

Health is a state of well-being. WHO defined it as 'State of complete physical, mental and social well-being and not merely the absence of disease and infirmity'.

Assessment (ANA) a systematic, dynamic process by which the nurse, through interaction with client, significant others and health care providers, collects and analyzes data about the client.

In the simple words, health assessment is collecting data about client health status. It is detailed study of the entire body in order to determine the general or mental condition of the body.

## PURPOSE OF HEALTH ASSESSMENT

1. To collect data about physical, mental and social well-being of client.
2. To identify the problem in early stage.
3. To determine the cause and extent of disease.
4. To evaluate, monitor the changes in client's health status (deterioration or improvement).
5. To determine the nature of treatment requirement for client.
6. To alleviate the complications.
7. To certify whether client is medically fit to resume duties.
8. To contribute to medical research.
9. To collect data systematically.
10. To compare the client's state of health with ideal state. Considering his age, gender, culture, physical, physiological and socio-economic status.

## HEALTH HISTORY

Health history is collecting in detail subjective data regarding client's health in a chronological order.

## PURPOSE OF HEALTH HISTORY

- To gather subjective data from client
- To develop nursing diagnosis
- To plan action for
  - promoting health
  - preventing disease
  - alleviating acute problem
  - minimize chronic health problem

- To meet client's expectation for health
- To compare client health status with optimum health.

## FACTORS AFFECTING THE COLLECTION OF SUBJECTIVE DATA

- Physical setting
- Client's personality and behavior
- Communication skill
- Problem
- Nurse's personality and behavior
- Nurse's knowledge and skill.

## FACTORS AFFECTING THE COLLECTION OF OBJECTIVE DATA

- Hearing
- Viewing
- Touching
- Tasting
- Smelling
- Thoroughness
- Knowledge
- Concentration
- Accurate technique
- Objectivity.

## ASSESSMENT OF NEWBORN

- **Introduction:** The healthy child represents the sound relation of physical, mental, social, psychological development and maintains a good balance among these variables of the life. Healthy child always belongs to the healthy environment or he is a symbol of healthy environment.
- **Definition of growth:** Growth is physical maturation resulting an increase in size or number of the body tissues and its various organs. It involves by multiplication of cell and an increase in intracellular substance. Growth changes of body can be measured in inch/cm and pound/kg. It is a progressive and measurable aspect of body.
- **Definition of development:** Development is the process of functional, physiological maturation of the body. Development is a progressive increase in skill and capacity to function. Development causes maturation and myelination of nervous system. It includes psychological, emotional and social changes. Development is qualitative aspect of maturation and difficult to measure the individual development.

### Stages of Growth and Development

The stages of growth and development are divided in intrauterine life or prenatal and extrauterine life or post- natal period.

**Prenatal period:**

| **Stage** | **Time period** |
|---|---|
| - Ovum | - 0 to 14 days after conception |
| - Embryo | - 14 days to 8 weeks |
| - Fetus | - 8 weeks to birth (8-40 weeks) |

**Postnatal period:**

Neonate/newborn

| | | |
|---|---|---|
| From birth to four weeks of life (0-28 days) | | |
| Infancy | - | First year of life (1 month-1 year) |
| Toddler | - | One to 3 years |
| Preschool child | - | 3 to 6 years (early childhood) |
| School-going child | - | 6 to 10 years (girls) |
| | - | 6 to 12 years (boy) (middle childhood) |
| Adolescent | - | From puberty to adulthood |
| Early adolescent | - | 12 – 14 years |
| Middle adolescent | - | 14 – 16 years |
| Late adolescent | - | 16 – 20 years |

# ADOLESCENT HEALTH

## INTRODUCTION

During the transition from childhood to adulthood, adolescents establish patterns of behavior and make lifestyle choices that affect both their current and future health. Adolescents and young adults are adversely affected by serious health and safety issues such as motor vehicle crashes, violence, substance use and sexual behavior. They also struggle to adapt behaviors that could decrease their risk of developing chronic diseases in adulthood—behaviors such as eating nutritiously, engaging in physical activity and choosing not to use tobacco. Environmental factors such as family, peer group, school and community characteristics also contribute to the challenges that adolescents face.

To have the most positive impact on adolescent health, government agencies, community organizations, schools and other community members must work together in a comprehensive approach. Providing safe and nurturing environments for our nation's youth can ensure that adolescents will be healthy and productive members of society.

## DEFINITION

According to WHO, the adolescent period is from the age of 10 to 19 years, i.e. the 2nd decade of life. It can be distinguished as early adolescence, age 10 to 13 years; middle adolescences—14 to 16 years; late adolescence— 17 to 20 years.

The period of youth is from 15 through 24 years. The adolescents and youth together are phrased as young people (10 to 24 years).

## GROWTH AND DEVELOPMENT

As the child moves from childhood to adolescence, he/she undergoes various physical, physiological, psychological and emotional changes, which are typical in adolescence.

### Physical Development

The physical changes, which occur in early adolescence include rapid increase in height, weight, muscles size and head and face size and it is known as adolescent growth spurt. The timing of the adolescent growth spurt varies in boys and girls and also within each sex. For girls the spurt in growth occurs about 2 years earlier to boys. In boys, it is between 13 to 15 years and in girls between 11 to 14 years.

### Physiological Development

Many endocrine glands contribute in rapid growth of adolescents. The most important glands are the pituitary glands and the sex glands. Pituitary gland is the master gland, because it secretes three gonadotropic hormones at puberty, which marks the beginning of the puberty. The gonadotropic hormones stimulate gonads to produce their own hormones. Androgen, the male sex hormone in boys, promotes the development of penis, the prostate gland, the seminal vesicles and secondary sex characteristics. Estrogen, the female sex hormone in girls, promotes the development of uterus, vagina, the fallopian tubes, breast, it also starts the menstrual cycle.

### Sexual Development

As the main impact is the production of gonadal hormones helps in the development of primary and secondary sexual characters in girls and boys at the time of puberty. In girls, reproductive system matures and gains in weight and size. About the age of 13 years menarche occurs. The secondary sex characteristics include growth of pubic hairs and hairs under arms, budding of the breast, change of voice, widening of hips, thighs become funnel shaped and broadening of shoulders.

In boys too, the male reproductive system matures and gains size and weight. The penis, prostate gland, the testes and scrotum are all enlarged at puberty. The secondary sexual characteristics are growth of pubic hairs and hair under arms, deepening of voice, widening of chest and shoulders, arms becoming more muscular, growth of hairs on face and body.

## Psychological Development

As the adolescent boys and girls grow in age, they mature mentally and emotionally. Even during early adolescence period, they develop capacity to apply principles of logic, to think critically in terms of theory, hypothesis, assumptions, etc. Emotionally, the adolescent boys and girls not only mature in physical intimacy with the opposite sex, but also in emotional intimacy, love and affection, etc. there are prompt sexual thoughts, day dreaming, heightened awareness of sexual attraction. In general, boys and girls become more interested in each other during puberty. Most of the adolescents experience frequent shifts in their mood because of hormonal adjustments, discomforts and concerns about the changes in their bodies.

It is, therefore, very important that the adolescents are helped in there proper growth and development. Attention should be given.

## HEALTH PROBLEMS DURING ADOLESCENCE

1. **Alcohol and drug use:** Alcohol is used by more young people in the United States than tobacco or illicit drugs. Excessive alcohol consumption is associated with approximately 75,000 deaths per year. Alcohol is a factor in approximately 41% of all deaths from motor vehicle crashes. Among youth, the use of alcohol and other drugs has also been linked to unintentional injuries, physical fights, academic and occupational problems, and illegal behavior.
2. **Nutrition:** Healthy eating is associated with reduced risk for many diseases, including the three leading causes of death: heart disease, cancer and stroke. Healthy eating in childhood and adolescence is important for proper growth and development and can prevent health problems such as obesity, dental caries and iron deficiency anemia. Most young people are not following the recommendations set forth in the Dietary Guidelines for Americans: of US youth aged 6 to 19, 67% exceed dietary guidelines recommendations for fat intake, 72% exceed recommendations for saturated fat intake. In 2007, only 21.4% of high school students reported eating fruits and vegetables five or more times daily (when fried potatoes and potato chips are excluded) during the past 7 days.
3. **Self-esteem related problems:** Self-esteem is closely identified with self-respect and identity. It implies proper regard for oneself as human being and an accurate sense of one's personal place within the large society of family, friends, associates and others. While lack of it can result in unworthiness. On the other hand low self-esteem, i.e. deficient sense of self, makes one unable to interact freely and responsibly with others at home, in school, at work place and in the society.

   To attain balanced self-esteem it is essential for adolescent to have:
   - Successful, accepted and satisfying relationship with parents, peers, teachers and others.
   - Acknowledge and respect qualities or attributes that make him/her special and different and that these qualities are approved by others;
   - Have power that comes from resources, opportunities and capability to influence the circumstances of his/her own life in important ways;
   - Have models that help him/her to establish meaningful values, goals, ideas and personal standards.
4. **Depression:** The occurrence of depression is related to adolescent's relationship to their parents, loosening of ties to their parents, family responsibilities, becoming independent, deviation in growth and development, etc.
5. **Tendency towards violence and accidents:** Adolescent, especially boys are very energetic at this age and are prone to road accidents because of fast and negligent driving. They are adventurous and are at particular risk of violent death due to greater risk taking and aggressive behavior. Homicides, suicides and accidents accounts for significant portion of all death in adolescents these days. Suicides and suicide attempts are associated with depression.
6. **Anorexia nervosa:** Anorexia nervosa occurs exclusively during adolescence or early adulthood. It is a rare psychological disturbance, which occurs more in girls than boys. Anorexia nervosa is also associated with unwillingness to assume an adult sexual role.
7. **Sexuality related problems:** Adolescent is the time when boys and girls are maturing sexually. They get attracted towards opposite sex. This is, but natural, to get feelings for each other. It is alright if there is no sexual exploitation. But because of

various prevailing conditions such as urbanization, moves towards nuclear family system, growth of slums, easy availability of pornographic material, exposure to seductive and exciting program of electronic media, loss of sociocultural values, etc.

The national crime record bureau had revealed the following information about violence against women:

- One act of eve-teasing every 51 minutes
- One rape every 54 minutes
- One kidnapping and abduction every 43 minutes
- One act of cruelty every 33 minutes
- One criminal offence against women every 7 minutes.

In India in 1997, of the 43 million reported cases of STD, majority of them acquired the disease during adolescence. Most of the injected drug users are the youth who get HIV infection through it. Because of liberal attitude towards sex, adolescent girls get pregnant during their teenage, i.e. before they are physically and mentally mature to bear children.

8. **Other problems:** These various problems/issues can be denoted as per acronym of **ADOLESCENT** as under:

**A.** Accidents, abortions, anemia, addiction, anxiety, academic stress.
**D.** Developing identity crises, depression leading to suicidal tendency, developmental issues (physical, hormonal, emotional, etc.)
**O.** Onset of puberty, onset of life-time habits.
**L.** Lack of correct health information, low self-esteem.
**E.** Experimentation and explorative nature, early marriage/child bearing and exploitation.
**S.** Sexual usage/abuse/violence, STDs including HIV/AIDS.
**C.** Clan spirit (peer group pressure), concern about body image.
**E.** Emotional turmoil.
**N.** Nutrition problem/neglect.
**T.** Teenage pregnancy, turmoils (emotional).

Facts about the teen-parent relationship during the teen years:

- Parent relationships are not necessarily undermined by peer relationships.
- While it seems that teens are influenced by their peers, parents continue to be the most influential factor in their lives.
- Parent-adolescent conflict increases between childhood and early adolescence; although in most families, its frequency and intensity remain low.
- Parents who continue to communicate with their teens, even when there are conflicts, actually maintain closer relationships.

## International Efforts

WHO reflected this in the establishment of the adolescent health program in 1990. This program was renamed to adolescent health and development program around 1996, to promote not only adolescent health, but also to promote physical, psychological and social development of adolescents of both sexes, which underlie their health behavior and relationships. In order to promote the health and development of young people between the ages of 10 and 24, WHO has advocated:

To expand the knowledge base of comprehensive adolescent health.

To formulate policy and program for adolescent health and developments based on up-to-date knowledge.

To develop and adopt methods, which would facilitate need-based actions.

Under this program more than 200 publications and documents in variety of languages have been produced. Two of the most important publications are "the health of young people: a challenge and a promise" and joint WHO/UNICEF: "a picture of health, A review and annotated bibliography of the health of young people in developing countries".

## National Efforts

As far adolescents sexual and reproductive health is concerned, it refers to physical and emotional well-being of adolescents and includes their ability to remain free from unwanted pregnancy, unsafe abortions, sexually transmitted disease including HIV/AIDS and all forms of sexual violence and coercion keeping in mind the needs of and problems, which are faced by adolescents as a result of their growth and development and transition from childhood to adulthood.

## HEALTH PROMOTION INTERVENTIONS

**Safe and supportive environment:** The safe and supportive environment not only includes hygienically physical environment, but also biological, psychosocial and spiritual environment. The environment should be safe and supportive at the family, neighborhood, community and at school level.

Personal hygiene and adoption of healthy lifestyle: It is very important for adolescents to maintain good personal hygiene. Both boys and girls should take daily bath; wear clean undergarments and clothes. The boys must form the habit of keeping their organ clean by retracting foreskin during bath and urination. The girls should use clean sanitary napkins during menstruation, which must be changed frequently.

Good nutrition and food hygiene: Adolescence is a period of rapid physical growth and more physical activities. Therefore both boys and girls require well-balanced nutritious diet to have normal growth and to keep fit. The adolescents should learn to relax and eat properly at meal time. They should avoid taking junk food. They should take wholesome snacks preferably made from groundnut, parched chana, etc. inadequate diet leads to malnutrition and results in various deficiencies disease, e.g. puberty goiter due to iodine deficiency, night blindness due to vitamin A deficiency, anemia due to lack of iron especially in girls.

**Sex education:** Adolescents generally are less informed, less experienced and less confident about sexual matters and get into a lot of sexual problems such as premarital unprotected sexual indulgence resulting in STDs, illegitimate teenage pregnancies, sexual abuse, violence, exploitation, etc. therefore, it is very important to conduct sex education for adolescents, so that they learn about: normal functioning of reproductive system, the healthy relationship with opposite sex, safe and protected sex, contraceptives, measures to prevent sexual exploitation by any one in the family, school/college, neighborhood, etc.

Gender sensitization; studies done in this area have revealed that there is discrimination in such areas as distribution of food in amount and quality, opportunities for education, skills training, employment, wages, health care, etc. the neglect of the girl child affects her health in many ways. They are malnourished, underweight, anemic, etc. they should be helped to develop logical thinking for providing opportunities on the basis of interest and choice and not on the basis of sex. Efforts must be put in to elevate gender-related prejudices among adolescents and create awareness about the importance of gender equality.

**Health education and communication:** They are not much informed, therefore-less confident about sex-related facts and issues and their abilities than adults. They do not have much information about the health services, which exist and are available to them. It is, therefore, important that good health education and communication program should be planned and organized for adolescents as part of school health program and school curriculum in which school administration and teacher should take active responsibility. Health personnel can give assistance and guidance.

Health education and communication program needs to be specially organized for adolescent as part of RCH program. It needs to be implemented at convenient location such as youth clubs, work sites, schools/colleges, clinics, etc. and at suitable timings. The environment must be friendly, comfortable and appropriate for all the adolescents. This way, it is accessible and motivating. It should include information on growth and development, nutrition, sexuality, personnel hygiene and lifestyle, substance abuse, utilization of health services.

**Counseling services:** Often adolescents require counseling services to deal with their individual problems, which they face during their period of development. The problems may be related to smoking, etc.; academic performance, etc. therefore need-based counseling services need to be provided at school, RCH clinics, drug addiction clinics, etc.

## COMMUNITY HEALTH NURSES ROLE AND RESPONSIBILITIES

The major responsibilities, which should be carried by community health nurse, are as under:

- Does health assessment using variety of tools and techniques to assess physical, mental/emotional and social health.
- Monitors growth and development, vital signs, immunization and nutrition status.
- Identifies deviations and abnormalities, health and nursing needs.
- Plans and implements comprehensive health and nursing care.
- Evaluates care given.
- Does education and counseling of adolescent, their parents and teachers in general, and about any deviation or abnormality in particular.

Seeks adolescent's participation by organizing them into youth clubs and health groups in meeting their health needs and dealing with their problems. She can make the use of her energies in various community activities.

# ASSIGNMENT–20 (A): PHYSICAL HEALTH ASSESSMENT FOR NEWBORN/INFANT

## I. Demographic Data

Age: ____________________

Date of birth: ____________________

Sex: ____________________

Classification: ____________________

Head of the family: ____________________

Address: ____________________

____________________

____________________

## II. Birth history

**Antenatal history**

Antenatal checkup: Yes/No
Immunization: Yes/No
Exposure to drug: ____________________
Viral infection: Yes/No

**Natal history**

Place of birth: Hospital/home
Mode of delivery: Normal/LSCS/instrumental
Gestation: Term/preterm/postmature
Delivery conducted by: Trained/untrained personnel
Condition at birth: active/asphyxiated/______
Congenital abnormalities: Yes/No
If yes, specify ____________________
Complication if any ____________________
Birth weight: ____________________

**Postnatal history**

BABY:

1. Birth injury Yes/No
2. Icterus Yes/No
3. Eye discharge Yes/No
4. Umbilical infection Yes/No

MOTHER:

Any complication ____________________

**Health History**

**Family health history**

____________________

____________________

____________________

____________________

____________________

**Past medical/surgical history**

______________________________________________________________________

______________________________________________________________________

______________________________________________________________________

______________________________________________________________________

**Present health history**

______________________________________________________________________

______________________________________________________________________

______________________________________________________________________

______________________________________________________________________

**III. Physical Assessment:**

1. **Vital sign** :Temperature ________, Heart rate _______, Respiration _________
2. **Head:**
   Fontanelle :Bulged/sunken/closed/normal
   Size :Microcephaly/hydrocephalus/normal
   Hair color :Flag sign/dry/thin/normal
   Distribution :Equal/partial/alopecia
   Dandruff :Present/absent
3. **Eyes**
   Eyebrows :Absent/present
   Eyelashes :Absent/present
   Follicle/sty :Absent/present
   Eyelids
   Edema :Absent/present
   Lesion :Absent/present
   Eyeballs :Protruded/sunken/normal conjunctiva
   Color :Pale/red/yellow tinged/blue tinged
   Cornea :Transparent/smooth/moist
   Visual acuity :Normal/myopia/hyperopia
   Eye movement :Normal/strabismus (squint)
   Blurred/double vision
4. **Polyps** :Absent/present
5. **Mouth and pharynx**
   a. Mucous membrane :Normal/red/swelling cyanosis
   b. Breath :Normal/halitosis
   c. Throat :Normal/sore throat/enlarged tonsils
   d. Gum :Normal/bleeding gum/gingivitis
   f. Tongue :Cyanotic/pale/moist/dry/coated/ulcers
   g. Oral hygienic habits :Habits Brushing---- times/day
   h. Material used :Brush/neem stick/fingers
   i. Dentifrice :Tooth powder/tooth paste/ash/mud
6. **Neck**
   lymph node :Enlarged/normal
   Thyroid gland :Normal/enlarged/midline/smooth/firm/non-tender
7. **Chest**
   Shape :Normal/barrel shaped/pigeon chest
   Chest movement :Symmetrical/asymmetrical
8. **Heart** :Position of the heart:right/left
   Heart sound :Normal/murmur/bruit

9. **Breasts**
   Size :Normal/abnormal-specify
   Position :Normal/abnormal
10. **Axillaries lymph nodes** :Palpable/non-palpable
11. **Abdomen**
    a. Skin :Rash/lesion/scars
    b. Umbilical:
    c. Peristalsis :Visible/not visible
    d. Size :Normal/abnormal
    e. Bowel sound :Absent/present
12. **Genitals**
    a. Scrotal swelling or mass :Absent/present
    b. Lymph nodes :Palpable/not palpable
13. **Lower extremities**
    a. Gait :Normal/abnormal
    b. Contour :Normal/locked knee
    c. Mobility: (Range of motion) :Normal/limited
14. **Integumentary system**
    a. Skin color : Normal/dark pigmented/smooth/soft/dry
    b. Temperature : Normal/cold/warm/dry
    c. Nails : Normal/blue/yellow/clubbing

## ANTHROPOMETRIC MEASUREMENT

Height/weight/HCC/CC/MAC ________________________________

Diet pattern: 24 hours recall

**Infants:**

Feeding: breast/artificial ________________________ times/day and night

Supplementary feeding ________________________ times/day and night

Weaning: ________________________ month

**Nutritional History**

| Food items | Cooked items | Raw amount | Calorie (K cal) | Proteins (g) | Fat | Calcium (mg) | Vitamin A | Iron |
|---|---|---|---|---|---|---|---|---|
| Breakfast<br>Midmorning<br>Lunch<br>Tea<br>Dinner | | | | | | | | |
| Total intake | | | | | | | | |
| Requirement | | | | | | | | |
| Excess/Deficit | | | | | | | | |

$$\text{Degree of malnutrition} = \frac{\text{Actual weight of the child}}{\text{Expected weight}} \times 10$$

## IV. Newborn Appraisals

| | |
|---|---|
| Sucking | Yes/No |
| Swallowing | Yes/No |
| Blinking | Yes/No |
| Rooting | Yes/No |
| Moro | Yes/No |
| Doll's eye | Yes/No |
| Startle | Yes/No |
| Tonic neck | Yes/No |
| Babinski | Yes/No |
| Stepping | Yes/No |

## V. Developmental Milestones: Growth and Development of Newborn/Infant

a. Biological development

| Physical development | Findings of baby | Expected |
|---|---|---|
| Labyrinth righting | | |
| Neck righting | | |
| Parachute reflex | | |
| Landau reflex | | |
| Dentition | | |
| Vital sign | | |

b. Sensory changes

| | Yes | No | Comment |
|---|---|---|---|
| i. Vision<br>• Follow range 90 degree<br>• Binocular vision<br>• Developed color preference<br>• Follows rapidly moving objects<br>ii. Hearing<br>• Turns head to side where sound made<br>• Imitates sounds<br>• Responds to own name | | | |

c. Motor Development

| | Yes | No | Comment |
|---|---|---|---|
| i. Fine motor development<br>• Desires to grasp<br>• Transfers object from one hand to another<br>• Explores movable parts of toy<br>ii. Gross motor development<br>1. Head control<br>• Able to lift the head and front position of the chest<br>• Able to raise the chest and upper part of the abdomen | | | |

| | Yes | No | Comment |
|---|---|---|---|
| 2. Rolling over<br>• Rolls from back to side<br>• Rolls from abdomen to back<br>• Rolls from back to abdomen<br>3. Sitting<br>• Sits with good head control with support<br>• Sits alone without support<br>4. Locomotion<br>• Moves from sitting to kneeling<br>• Crawls with abdomen on floor<br>• Stands holding onto furniture | | | |

d. Cognitive development

| | Yes | No | Comment |
|---|---|---|---|
| Sensory motor phase<br>1. Use of reflex<br>• Sucking and swallowing<br>2. Primary circular reaction<br>• Recognizes stimulus that produces a response<br>• Engages in activity for the pleasure<br>• Recognizes orderly sequence of an event<br>3. Secondary circulation reaction<br>• Recognizes symbol<br>• Imitates sound<br>4. Co-ordination of secondary schemes and their applications to new situations<br>• Associates symbol with events<br>• Distinguishes objects from related activity<br>• Has concept of object permanence | | | |

e. Social development

| | Yes | No | Comment |
|---|---|---|---|
| • Recognizes parents<br>• Has fear of strangers<br>• Holds arms out to be picked up<br>• Imitates others<br>• Has definite likes and dislikes<br>• Searches for dropped objects | | | |

f. Language

| | Yes | No | Comment |
|---|---|---|---|
| • Imitates sounds<br>• Laughs aloud<br>• Takes pleasure in hearing over sounds<br>• Comprehends meaning to simple words<br>• Obeys simple commands and responds to that name | | | |

g. Play

| | Yes | No | Comment |
|---|---|---|---|
| • Plays alone<br>• Plays with toys | | | |

## VI. Immunization

| Vaccine | At birth | 1 | 2 | 3 | 4 | 5 | 1st Booster | 2nd Booster |
|---|---|---|---|---|---|---|---|---|
| BCG | | | | | | | | |
| DPT | | | | | | | | |
| OPV | | | | | | | | |
| Measles | | | | | | | | |
| Hepatitis B | | | | | | | | |
| TT | | | | | | | | |
| MMR | | | | | | | | |
| Others | | | | | | | | |

## VII. Health Teaching

## VIII. Summary

# ASSIGNMENT–20 (B): PHYSICAL HEALTH ASSESSMENT FOR NEWBORN/INFANT

## I. Demographic Data

Age: ____________________

Date of birth: ____________________

Sex: ____________________

Classification: ____________________

Head of the family: ____________________

Address: ____________________

____________________

____________________

## II. Birth History

**Antenatal history**

Antenatal checkup: Yes/No
Immunization: Yes/No
Exposure to drug: ____________________
Viral infection: Yes/No

**Natal history**

Place of birth: Hospital/home
Mode of delivery: Normal/LSCS/instrumental
Gestation: Term/preterm/postmature
Delivery conducted by: Trained/untrained personnel
Condition at birth: Active/asphyxiated/______
Congenital abnormalities: Yes/No
If yes, specify ____________________
Complication, if any ____________________
Birth weight: ____________________

**Postnatal history**

BABY:

1. Birth injury Yes/No
2. Icterus Yes/No
3. Eye discharge Yes/No
4. Umbilical infection Yes/No

MOTHER:
Any complication ____________________

### Health History

**Family health history**

____________________

____________________

____________________

____________________

____________________

**Past medical/surgical history**

______________________________________________
______________________________________________
______________________________________________
______________________________________________
______________________________________________

**Present health history**

______________________________________________
______________________________________________
______________________________________________
______________________________________________
______________________________________________

**III. Physical Assessment**

1. **Vital sign** :Temperature ______, Heart rate ______, Respiration ______
2. **Head**
   - Fontanelle :Bulged/sunken/closed/normal
   - Size :Microcephaly/hydrocephalus/normal
   - Hair color :Flag sign/dry/thin/normal
   - Distribution :Equal/partial/alopecia
   - Dandruff :Present/absent
3. **Eyes**
   - Eyebrows :Absent/present
   - Eyelashes :Absent/present
   - Follicle/sty :Absent/present
   - Eyelids
   - Edema :Absent/present
   - Lesion :Absent/present
   - Eyeballs :Protruded/sunken/normal conjunctiva
   - Color :Pale/red/yellow tinged/blue tinged
   - Cornea :Transparent/smooth/moist
   - Visual acuity :Normal/myopia/hyperopia
   - Eye movement :Normal/strabismus(squint) Blurred/double vision
4. **Polyps** :Absent/present
5. **Mouth and pharynx**
   a. Mucous membrane :Normal/red/swelling cyanosis
   b. Breath :Normal/halitosis
   c. Throat :Normal/sore throat/enlarged tonsils
   d. Gum :Normal/bleeding gum/gingivitis
   e. Tongue :Cyanotic/pale/moist/dry/coated/ulcers
   f. Oral hygienic habits :Brushing ______ times/day
   g. Material used :Brush/neem stick/fingers
   h. Dentifrices :Tooth powder/tooth paste/ash/mud
6. **Neck**
   - Lymph node :Enlarged/normal
   - Thyroid gland :Normal/enlarged/midline/smooth/firm/non-tender

7. **Chest**
   Shape :Normal/barrel shaped/pigeon chest
   Chest movement :Symmetrical/asymmetrical
8. **Heart:** (Position of the heart) :Right/left
   Heart sound :Normal/murmur/bruit
9. **Breasts**
   Size :Normal/abnormal-specify
   Position :Normal/abnormal
10. **Axillaries lymph nodes** :Palpable/non-palpable
11. **Abdomen**
    a. Skin :Rash/lesion/scars/
    b. Umbilical :
    c. Peristalsis :Visible/not visible
    d. Size :Normal/abnormal
    e. Bowel sound :Absent/present
12. **Genitals**
    a. Scrotal swelling or mass :Absent/present
    b. Lymph nodes :Palpable/not palpable
13. **Lower extremities:**
    a. Gait :Normal/abnormal
    b. Contour :Normal/locked knee
    c. Mobility :Range of motion:normal/limited
14. **Integumentary system**
    a. Skin color :Normal/dark pigmented/smooth/soft/dry
    b. Temperature :Normal/cold/warm/dry
    c. Nails :Normal/blue/yellow/clubbing

## ANTHROPOMETRIC MEASUREMENT

Height/weight/HCC/CC/MAC

______________________________

Diet pattern: 24 hours recall

**Infants:**

Feeding: Breast/artificial ____________ times/day and night

Supplementary feeding ____________ times/day and night

Weaning: ____________ month

**Nutritional History**

| Food items | Cooked items | Raw amount | Calorie (K cal) | Proteins (g) | Fat | Calcium (mg) | Vitamin A | Iron |
|---|---|---|---|---|---|---|---|---|
| Breakfast<br>Midmorning<br>Lunch<br>Tea<br>Dinner | | | | | | | | |
| Total intake | | | | | | | | |
| Requirement | | | | | | | | |
| Excess/deficit | | | | | | | | |

$$\text{Degree of malnutrition} = \frac{\text{Actual weight of the child}}{\text{Expected weight}} \times 10$$

**IV. Newborn Appraisals:**

| | |
|---|---|
| Sucking | Yes/No |
| Swallowing | Yes/No |
| Blinking | Yes/No |
| Rooting | Yes/No |
| Moro | Yes/No |
| Doll's eye | Yes/No |
| Startle | Yes/No |
| Tonic neck | Yes/No |
| Babinski | Yes/No |
| Stepping | Yes/No |

**V. DEVELOPMENTAL MILESTONES: GROWTH AND DEVELOPMENT OF NEWBORN/INFANT**

a. Biological development

| Physical development | Findings of baby | Expected |
|---|---|---|
| Labyrinth righting | | |
| Neck righting | | |
| Parachute reflex | | |
| Landau reflex | | |
| Dentition | | |
| Vital sign | | |

b. Sensory changes

| | Yes | No | Comment |
|---|---|---|---|
| i. Vision<br>• Follows range 90 degree<br>• Binocular vision<br>• Developed color preference<br>• Follows rapidly moving objects<br>ii. Hearing<br>• Turns head to side where sound made<br>• Imitates sounds<br>• Responds to own name | | | |

c. Motor development

| | Yes | No | Comment |
|---|---|---|---|
| i. Fine motor development<br>• Desires to grasp<br>• Transfers object from one hand to another<br>• Explores movable parts of toy<br>ii. Gross motor development<br>1. Head control<br>• Able to lift the head and front position of the chest<br>• Able to raise the chest and upper part of the abdomen<br>2. Rolling over<br>• Rolls from back to side<br>• Rolls from abdomen to back<br>• Rolls from back to abdomen | | | |

*Contd...*

*Contd...*

| | Yes | No | Comment |
|---|---|---|---|
| 3. Sitting<br>• Sits with good head control with support<br>• Sits alone without support<br>4. Locomotion<br>• Moves from sitting to kneeling<br>• Crawls with abdomen on floor<br>• Stands holding onto furniture | | | |

d. Cognitive development

| | Yes | No | Comment |
|---|---|---|---|
| Sensory Motor Phase<br>1. Use of reflex<br>• Sucking and swallowing<br>2. Primary circular reaction<br>• Recognizes stimulus that produces a response<br>• Engages in activity for the pleasure<br>• Recognizes orderly sequence of an event<br>3. Secondary circulation reaction<br>• Recognizes symbol<br>• Imitates sound<br>4. Co-ordination of secondary schemes and their applications to new situations<br>• Associates symbol with events<br>• Distinguishes objects from related activity<br>• Has concept of object permanence | | | |

e. Social development

| | Yes | No | Comment |
|---|---|---|---|
| • Recognizes parents<br>• Has fear of strangers<br>• Holds arms out to be picked up<br>• Imitates others<br>• Has definite likes and dislikes<br>• Searches for dropped objects | | | |

f. Language

| | Yes | No | Comment |
|---|---|---|---|
| • Imitates sounds<br>• Laughs aloud<br>• Takes pleasure in hearing over sounds<br>• Comprehends meaning to simple words<br>• Obeys simple commands and responds to that name | | | |

g. Play

| | Yes | No | Comment |
|---|---|---|---|
| • Plays alone<br>• Plays with toys | | | |

## VI. Immunization

| Vaccine | At birth | 1 | 2 | 3 | 4 | 5 | 1st booster | 2nd booster |
|---|---|---|---|---|---|---|---|---|
| BCG | | | | | | | | |
| DPT | | | | | | | | |
| OPV | | | | | | | | |
| Measles | | | | | | | | |
| Hepatitis B | | | | | | | | |
| TT | | | | | | | | |
| MMR | | | | | | | | |
| Others | | | | | | | | |

## VII. Health Teaching

## VIII. Summary

# ASSIGNMENT–20 (C) : PHYSICAL HEALTH ASSESSMENT FOR NEWBORN/INFANT

## I. Demographic Data

Age: ____________________

Date of birth: ____________________

Sex: ____________________

Classification: ____________________

Head of the family: ____________________

Address: ____________________

____________________

## II. Birth History

**Antenatal history**

Antenatal checkup: Yes/No

Immunization: Yes/No

Exposure to drug: ____________________

Viral infection: Yes/No

**Natal history**

Place of birth: hospital/home

Mode of delivery: normal/LSCS/instrumental

Gestation: Term/preterm/postmature

Delivery conducted by: Trained/untrained personnel

Condition at birth: active/asphyxiated/__________

Congenital abnormalities: Yes/No

If yes, specify ____________________

Complication, if any ____________________

Birth weight: ____________________

**Postnatal history:**

BABY:

1. Birth injury Yes/No
2. Icterus Yes/No
3. Eye discharge Yes/No
4. Umbilical infection Yes/No

MOTHER:

Any complication ____________________

## Health History

**Family health history**

____________________

____________________

____________________

____________________

____________________

**Past medical/surgical history**

______________________________________________________________________

______________________________________________________________________

______________________________________________________________________

______________________________________________________________________

**Present health history**

______________________________________________________________________

______________________________________________________________________

______________________________________________________________________

______________________________________________________________________

**III. Physical Assessment**

1. **Vital sign** :Temperature ________, Heart rate ________, Respiration ________
2. **Head**
   - Fontanelle :Bulged/sunken/closed/normal
   - Size :Microcephaly/hydrocephalus/normal
   - Hair color :Flag sign/dry/thin/normal
   - Distribution :Equal/partial/alopecia
   - Dandruff :Present/absent
3. **Eyes**
   - Eyebrows :Absent/present
   - Eyelashes :Absent/present
   - Follicle/sty :Absent/present
   - Eyelids
   - Edema :Absent/present
   - Lesion :Absent/present
   - Eyeballs :Protruded/sunken/normal conjunctiva
   - Color :Pale/red/yellow tinged/blue tinged
   - Cornea :Transparent/smooth/moist
   - Visual acuity :Normal/myopia/hyperopia
   - Eye movement :Normal/strabismus (squint)
   - Blurred/double vision :Absent/present
4. **Polyps**
5. **Mouth and pharynx**
   - a. Mucous membrane :Normal/red/swelling cyanosis
   - b. Breath :Normal/halitosis
   - c. Throat :Normal/sore throat/enlarged tonsils
   - d. Gum :Normal/bleeding gum/gingivitis
   - f. Tongue :Cyanotic/pale/moist/dry/coated/ulcers
   - g. Oral hygienic habits :Brushing---- times/day
   - h. Material used :Brush/neem stick/fingers
   - i. Dentifrices :Tooth powder/toothpaste/ash/mud
6. **Neck**
   - Lymph node :Enlarged/normal
   - Thyroid gland :Normal/enlarged/mid line/smooth/firm/non-tender
7. **Chest**
   - Shape :Normal/barrel shaped/pigeon chest
   - Chest movement :Symmetrical/asymmetrical

8. **Heart**
   Position of the heart :Right/left
   Heart sound :Normal/murmur/bruit
9. **Breasts**
   Size :Normal/abnormal-specify
   Position :Normal/abnormal
10. **Axillaries lymph nodes** :Palpable/non-palpable
11. **Abdomen**
    a. Skin :Rash/lesion/scars/
    b. Umbilical
    c. Peristalsis :Visible/not visible
    d. Size :Normal/abnormal
    e. Bowel sound :Absent/present
12. **Genitals**
    a. Scrotal swelling or mass :Absent/present
    b. Lymph nodes :Palpable/not palpable
13. **Lower extremities:**
    a. Gait :Normal/abnormal
    b. Contour :Normal/locked knee
    c. Mobility :Range of motion:normal/limited
14. **Integumentary system**
    a. Skin color :Normal/dark pigmented/smooth/soft/dry
    b. Temperature :Normal/cold/warm/dry
    c. Nails :Normal/blue/yellow/clubbing

## ANTHROPOMETRIC MEASUREMENT

Height/weight/HCC/CC/MAC

____________________________________________

Diet pattern: 24 hours recall
Infants:
Feeding: Breast/artificial ____________________ times/day and night
Supplementary feeding ____________________ times/day and night
Weaning: ____________________ month

## Nutritional History

| Food items | Cooked items | Raw amount | Calorie (K cal) | Proteins (g) | Fat | Calcium (mg) | Vitamin A | Iron |
|---|---|---|---|---|---|---|---|---|
| Breakfast<br>Midmorning<br>Lunch<br>Tea<br>Dinner | | | | | | | | |
| Total intake | | | | | | | | |
| Requirement | | | | | | | | |
| Excess/deficit | | | | | | | | |

$$\text{Degree of malnutrition} = \frac{\text{Actual weight of the child}}{\text{Expected weight}} \times 10$$

**IV. Newborn Appraisals:**

| | |
|---|---|
| Sucking | Yes/No |
| Swallowing | Yes/No |
| Blinking | Yes/No |
| Rooting | Yes/No |
| Moro | Yes/No |
| Doll's eye | Yes/No |
| Startle | Yes/No |
| Tonic neck | Yes/No |
| Babinski | Yes/No |
| Stepping | Yes/No |

**V. Developmental milestones: Growth and development of newborn/infant**

a. Biological development

| Physical development | Findings of baby | Expected |
|---|---|---|
| Labyrinth righting<br>Neck righting<br>Parachute reflex<br>Landau reflex<br>Dentition<br>Vital sign | | |

b. Sensory changes

| | Yes | No | Comment |
|---|---|---|---|
| i. Vision<br>• Follows range 90 degree<br>• Binocular vision<br>• Developed color preference<br>• Follows rapidly moving objects<br>ii. Hearing<br>• Turns head to side where sound made<br>• Imitates sounds<br>• Responds to own name | | | |

c. Motor development

| | Yes | No | Comment |
|---|---|---|---|
| i. Fine motor development<br>• Desires to grasp<br>• Transfers object from one hand to another<br>• Explores movable parts of toy<br>ii. Gross motor development<br>1. Head control<br>• Able to lift the head and front position of the chest<br>• Able to raise the chest and upper part of the abdomen<br>2. Rolling over<br>• Rolls from back to side<br>• Rolls from abdomen to back<br>• Rolls from back to abdomen | | | |

*Contd...*

*Contd...*

| | Yes | No | Comment |
|---|---|---|---|
| 3. Sitting<br>• Sits with good head control with support<br>• Sits alone without support<br>4. Locomotion<br>• Moves from sitting to kneeling<br>• Crawls with abdomen on floor<br>• Stands holding on to furniture | | | |

d. Cognitive development

| | Yes | No | Comment |
|---|---|---|---|
| Sensory Motor Phase<br>1. Use of reflex<br>• Sucking and swallowing<br>2. Primary circular reaction<br>• Recognizes stimulus that produces a response<br>• Engages in activity for the pleasure<br>• Recognizes orderly sequence of an event<br>3. Secondary circulation reaction<br>• Recognizes symbol<br>• Imitates sound<br>4. Coordination of secondary schemes and their applications to new situations<br>• Associates symbol with events<br>• Distinguishes objects from related activity<br>• Has concept of object permanence | | | |

e. Social development

| | Yes | No | Comment |
|---|---|---|---|
| • Recognizes parents<br>• Has fear of strangers<br>• Holds arms out to be picked up<br>• Imitates others<br>• Has definite likes and dislikes<br>• Searches for dropped objects | | | |

f. Language

| | Yes | No | Comment |
|---|---|---|---|
| • Imitates sounds<br>• Laughs aloud<br>• Takes pleasure in hearing over sounds<br>• Comprehends meaning to simple words<br>• Obeys simple commands and responds to that name | | | |

g. Play

| | Yes | No | Comment |
|---|---|---|---|
| • Plays alone<br>• Plays with toys | | | |

## VI. Immunization

| Vaccine | At birth | 1 | 2 | 3 | 4 | 5 | 1st booster | 2nd booster |
|---|---|---|---|---|---|---|---|---|
| BCG | | | | | | | | |
| DPT | | | | | | | | |
| OPV | | | | | | | | |
| Measles | | | | | | | | |
| Hepatitis B | | | | | | | | |
| TT | | | | | | | | |
| MMR | | | | | | | | |
| Others | | | | | | | | |

## VII. Health Teaching

## VIII. Summary

# ASSIGNMENT–20 (D): PHYSICAL HEALTH ASSESSMENT FOR NEWBORN/INFANT

## I. Demographic Data

Age: __________

Date of birth: __________

Sex: __________

Classification: __________

Head of the family: __________

Address: __________

## II. Birth History

**Antenatal history**

Antenatal checkup: Yes/No

Immunization: Yes/No

Exposure to drug: __________

Viral infection: Yes/No

**Natal history**

Place of birth: Hospital/home

Mode of delivery: Normal/LSCS/instrumental

Gestation: Term/preterm/postmature

Delivery conducted by: Trained/untrained personnel

Condition at birth: Active/asphyxiated/__________

Congenital abnormalities: Yes/No

If yes, specify __________

Complication if any __________

Birth weight: __________

**Postnatal history:**

BABY:

1. Birth injury Yes/No
2. Icterus Yes/No
3. Eye discharge Yes/No
4. Umbilical infection Yes/No

MOTHER:

Any complication __________

**Health History**

**Family health history**

__________

**Past medical/surgical history**

______________________________________________________________________
______________________________________________________________________
______________________________________________________________________
______________________________________________________________________
______________________________________________________________________
______________________________________________________________________

**Present health history**

______________________________________________________________________
______________________________________________________________________
______________________________________________________________________
______________________________________________________________________
______________________________________________________________________
______________________________________________________________________

**III. Physical Assessment**

1. **Vital sign** :Temperature ________, Heart rate ________, Respiration ________
2. **Head**
   - Fontanelle :Bulged/sunken/closed/normal
   - Size :Microcephaly/hydrocephalus/normal
   - Hair color :Flag sign/dry/thin/normal
   - Distribution :Equal/partial/alopecia
   - Dandruff :Present/absent
3. **Eyes**
   - Eyebrows :Absent/present
   - Eyelashes :Absent/present
   - Follicle/sty :Absent/present
   - Eyelids
   - Edema :Absent/present
   - Lesion :Absent/present
   - Eyeballs :Protruded/sunken/normal conjunctiva
   - Color :Pale/red/yellow tinged/blue tinged
   - Cornea :Transparent/smooth/moist
   - Visual acuity :Normal/myopia/hyperopia
   - Eye movement :Normal/strabismus (squint)
   - Blurred/double vision
4. **Polyps** :Absent/present
5. **Mouth and pharynx**
   - a. Mucous membrane :Normal/red/swelling cyanosis
   - b. Breath :Normal/halitosis
   - c. Throat :Normal/sore throat/enlarged tonsils
   - d. Gum :Normal/bleeding gum/gingivitis
   - f. Tongue :Cyanotic/pale/moist/dry/coated/ulcers
   - g. Oral hygienic habits :Brushing ________ times/day
   - h. Material used :Brush/neem stick/fingers
   - i. Dentifrices :Tooth powder/toothpaste/ash/mud
6. **Neck**
   - Lymph node :Enlarged/normal
   - Thyroid gland :Normal/enlarged/midline/smooth/firm/non-tender

7. **Chest**
   Shape :Normal/barrel shaped/pigeon chest
   Chest movement :Symmetrical/asymmetrical
8. **Heart**
   Position of the heart :Right/left
   Heart sound :Normal/murmur/bruit
9. **Breasts**
   Size :Normal/abnormal-specify
   position :Normal/abnormal
10. **Axillaries lymph nodes** :Palpable/non palpable
11. **Abdomen**
    a. Skin :Rash/lesion/scars/
    b. Umbilical :
    c. Peristalsis :Visible/not visible
    d. Size :Normal/abnormal
    e. Bowel sound :Absent/present
12. **Genitals**
    a. Scrotal swelling or mass :Absent/present
    b. Lymph nodes :Palpable/not palpable
13. **Lower extremities**
    a. Gait: Normal/abnormal
    b. Contour: Normal/locked knee
    c. Mobility: (Range of motion): normal/limited
14. **Integumentary system**
    a. Skin color : Normal/dark pigmented/smooth/soft/dry
    b. Temperature : Normal/cold/warm/dry
    c. Nails : Normal/blue/yellow/clubbing

## ANTHROPOMETRIC MEASUREMENT

Height/weight/HCC/CC/MAC

_______________________________________________

Diet pattern: 24 hours recall
**Infants:**
Feeding: Breast/artificial ____________________ times/day and night
Supplementary feeding ____________________ times/day and night
Weaning: ____________________ month

## Nutritional History

| Food items | Cooked items | Raw amount | Calorie | Proteins (g) | Fat | Calcium (mg) | Vitamin A | Iron |
|---|---|---|---|---|---|---|---|---|
| Breakfast<br>Midmorning<br>Lunch<br>Tea<br>Dinner | | | | | | | | |
| Total intake | | | | | | | | |
| Requirement | | | | | | | | |
| Excess/deficit | | | | | | | | |

$$\text{Degree of malnutrition} = \frac{\text{Actual weight of the child}}{\text{Expected weight}} \times 10$$

## IV. Newborn Appraisals

| | |
|---|---|
| Sucking | Yes/No |
| Swallowing | Yes/No |
| Blinking | Yes/No |
| Rooting | Yes/No |
| Moro | Yes/No |
| Doll's eye | Yes/No |
| Startle | Yes/No |
| Tonic neck | Yes/No |
| Babinski | Yes/No |
| Stepping | Yes/No |

## V. Developmental Milestones: Growth and Development of Newborn/Infant

a. Biological development

| Physical development | Findings of baby | Expected |
|---|---|---|
| Labyrinth righting | | |
| Neck righting | | |
| Parachute reflex | | |
| Landau reflex | | |
| Dentition | | |
| Vital sign | | |

b. Sensory changes

| | Yes | No | Comment |
|---|---|---|---|
| i. Vision<br>• Follows range 90 degree<br>• Binocular vision<br>• Develops color preference<br>• Follows rapidly moving objects<br>ii. Hearing<br>• Turns head to side where sound made<br>• Imitates sounds<br>• Responds to own name | | | |

c. Motor development

| | Yes | No | Comment |
|---|---|---|---|
| i. Fine motor development<br>• Desires to grasp<br>• Transfers object from one hand to another<br>• Explores movable parts of toy<br>ii. Gross motor development<br>1. Head control<br>• Able to lift the head and front position of the chest<br>• Able to raise the chest and upper part of the abdomen<br>2. Rolling over<br>• Rolls from back to side<br>• Rolls from abdomen to back<br>• Rolls from back to abdomen | | | |

*Contd...*

*Contd...*

| | Yes | No | Comment |
|---|---|---|---|
| 3. Sitting<br>• Sits with good head control with support<br>• Sits alone without support<br>4. Locomotion<br>• Moves from sitting top kneeling<br>• Crawls with abdomen on floor<br>• Stands holding onto furniture | | | |

d. Cognitive development

| | Yes | No | Comment |
|---|---|---|---|
| Sensory Motor Phase<br>1. Use of reflex<br>• Sucking and swallowing<br>2. Primary circular reaction<br>• Recognizes stimulus that produces a response<br>• Engages in activity for the pleasure<br>• Recognizes orderly sequence of an event<br>3. Secondary circulation reaction<br>• Recognizes symbol<br>• Imitates sound<br>4. Coordination of secondary schemes and their applications to new situations<br>• Associates symbol with events<br>• Distinguishes objects from related activity<br>• Has concept of object permanence | | | |

e. Social development

| | Yes | No | Comment |
|---|---|---|---|
| • Recognizes parents<br>• Has fear of strangers<br>• Holds arms out to be picked up<br>• Imitates others<br>• Has definite likes and dislikes<br>• Searches for dropped objects | | | |

f. Language

| | Yes | No | Comment |
|---|---|---|---|
| • Imitates sounds<br>• Laughs aloud<br>• Takes pleasure in hearing over sounds<br>• Comprehends meaning to simple words<br>• Obeys simple commands and responds to that name | | | |

g. Play

| | Yes | No | Comment |
|---|---|---|---|
| • Plays alone<br>• Plays with toys | | | |

## VI. Immunization

| Vaccine | At birth | 1 | 2 | 3 | 4 | 5 | 1st booster | 2nd booster |
|---|---|---|---|---|---|---|---|---|
| BCG | | | | | | | | |
| DPT | | | | | | | | |
| OPV | | | | | | | | |
| Measles | | | | | | | | |
| Hepatitis B | | | | | | | | |
| TT | | | | | | | | |
| MMR | | | | | | | | |
| Others | | | | | | | | |

## VII. Health Teaching

## VIII. Summary

# ASSIGNMENT–20 (E): PHYSICAL HEALTH ASSESSMENT FOR NEWBORN/INFANT

## I. Demographic Data

Age: ____________________

Date of birth: ____________________

Sex: ____________________

Classification: ____________________

Head of the family: ____________________

Address: ____________________

____________________

## II. Birth History

**Antenatal history**

Antenatal checkup: Yes/No

Immunization: Yes/No

Exposure to drug: ____________________

Viral infection: Yes/No

**Natal history**

Place of birth: Hospital/Home

Mode of delivery: Normal/LSCS/Instrumental

Gestation: Term/Preterm/Postmature

Delivery conducted by: Trained/Untrained Personnel

Condition at birth: Active/Asphyxiated/________

Congenital abnormalities: Yes/No

If yes, specify ____________________

Complication if any ____________________

Birth weight: ____________________

**Postnatal history**

BABY:

1. Birth injury Yes/No
2. Icterus Yes/No
3. Eye discharge Yes/No
4. Umbilical infection Yes/No

MOTHER:

Any complication ____________________

## Health History

**Family health history**

____________________

____________________

____________________

____________________

____________________

____________________

**Past medical/surgical history**

___________________________________________

___________________________________________

___________________________________________

___________________________________________

**Present health history**

___________________________________________

___________________________________________

___________________________________________

___________________________________________

### III. Physical Assessment

1. **Vital sign** :Temperature ____________, Heart rate ____________, Respiration ____________
2. **Head** :
   - Fontanelle :Bulged/sunken/closed/normal
   - Size :Microcephaly/hydrocephalus/normal
   - Hair color :Flag sign/dry/thin/normal
   - Distribution :Equal/partial/alopecia
   - Dandruff :Present/absent
3. **Eyes**
   - Eyebrows :Absent/present
   - Eyelashes :Absent/present
   - Follicle/sty :Absent/present
   - Eyelids
   - Edema :Absent/present
   - Lesion :Absent/present
   - Eyeballs :Protruded/sunken/normal conjunctiva
   - Color :Pale/red/yellow tinged/blue tinged
   - Cornea :Transparent/smooth/moist
   - Visual acuity :Normal/myopia/hyperopia
   - Eye movement :Normal/strabismus (squint)
     Blurred/double vision
4. **Polyps** :Absent/present
5. **Mouth and pharynx**
   - a. Mucous membrane :Normal/red/swelling cyanosis
   - b. Breath :Normal/halitosis
   - c. Throat :Normal/sore throat/enlarged tonsils
   - d. Gum :Normal/bleeding gum/gingivitis
   - f. Tongue :Cyanotic/pale/moist/dry/coated/ulcers
   - g. Oral hygienic habits :Brushing ________ times/day
   - h. Material used :Brush/neem stick/fingers
   - i. Dentifrices :Tooth powder/tooth paste/ash/mud
6. **Neck**
   - Lymph node :Enlarged/normal
   - Thyroid gland :Normal/enlarged/midline/smooth/firm/non-tender
7. **Chest**
   - Shape :Normal/barrel shaped/pigeon chest
   - Chest movement :Symmetrical/asymmetrical

8. **Heart**
   Position of the heart :Right/left
   Heart sound :Normal/murmur/Bruit
9. **Breasts**
   Size :Normal/abnormal-specify
   Position :Normal/abnormal
10. **Axillaries lymph nodes** :Palpable/non-palpable
11. **Abdomen**
    a. Skin :Rash/lesion/scars/
    b. Umbilical :
    c. Peristalsis :Visible/not visible
    d. Size :Normal/abnormal
    e. Bowel sound :Absent/present
12. **Genitals**
    a. Scrotal swelling or mass :Absent/present
    b. Lymph nodes :Palpable/not palpable
13. **Lower extremities** :
    a. Gait :Normal/abnormal
    b. Contour: Normal/locked knee
    c. Mobility: (Range of motion) :Normal/limited
14. **Integumentary system**
    a. Skin color :Normal/dark pigmented/smooth/soft/dry
    b. Temperature :Normal/cold/warm/dry
    c. Nails :Normal/blue/yellow/clubbing

## ANTHROPOMETRIC MEASUREMENT

Height/weight/HCC/CC/MAC

______________________________

Diet pattern : 24 hours recall

**Infants:**

Feeding: Breast/artificial ____________________ times/day and night

Supplementary feeding ____________________ times/day and night

Weaning: ____________________ month

## Nutritional History

| Food items | Cooked items | Raw amount | Calorie (k cal) | Proteins (g) | Fat | Calcium (mg) | Vitamin A | Iron |
|---|---|---|---|---|---|---|---|---|
| Breakfast<br>Midmorning<br>Lunch<br>Tea<br>Dinner | | | | | | | | |
| Total intake | | | | | | | | |
| Requirement | | | | | | | | |
| Excess/deficit | | | | | | | | |

$$\text{Degree of malnutrition} = \frac{\text{Actual weight of the child}}{\text{Expected weight}} \times 10$$

## IV. Newborn Appraisals

| | |
|---|---|
| Sucking | Yes/No |
| Swallowing | Yes/No |
| Blinking | Yes/No |
| Rooting | Yes/No |
| Moro | Yes/No |
| Doll's eye | Yes/No |
| Startle | Yes/No |
| Tonic neck | Yes/No |
| Babinski | Yes/No |
| Stepping | Yes/No |

## V. Developmental Milestones: Growth and Development of Newborn/Infant

a. Biological development

| Physical development | Findings of baby | Expected |
|---|---|---|
| Labyrinth righting | | |
| Neck righting | | |
| Parachute reflex | | |
| Landau reflex | | |
| Dentition | | |
| Vital sign | | |

b. Sensory changes

| | Yes | No | Comment |
|---|---|---|---|
| i. Vision<br>• Follows range 90 degree<br>• Binocular vision<br>• Develops color preference<br>• Follows rapidly moving objects<br>ii. Hearing<br>• Turns head to side where sound made<br>• Imitates sounds<br>• Responds to own name | | | |

c. Motor development

| | Yes | No | Comment |
|---|---|---|---|
| i. Fine motor development<br>• Desires to grasp<br>• Transfers object from one hand to another<br>• Explores movable parts of toy<br>ii. Gross motor development<br>1. Head control<br>– Able to lift the head and front position of the chest<br>– Able to raise the chest and upper part of the abdomen<br>2. Rolling over<br>– Rolls from back to side<br>– Rolls from abdomen to back<br>– Rolls from back to abdomen | | | |

*Contd...*

*Contd...*

| | Yes | No | Comment |
|---|---|---|---|
| 3. Sitting<br>– Sits with good head control with support<br>– Sits alone without support<br>4. Locomotion<br>– Moves from sitting to kneeling<br>– Crawls with abdomen on floor<br>– Stands holding onto furniture | | | |

d. Cognitive development

| | Yes | No | Comment |
|---|---|---|---|
| Sensory Motor Phase<br>1. Use of reflex<br>• Sucking and swallowing<br>2. Primary circular reaction<br>• Recognizes stimulus that produces a response<br>• Engages in activity for the pleasure<br>• Recognizes orderly sequence of an event<br>3. Secondary circulation reaction<br>• Recognizes symbol<br>• Imitates sound<br>4. Coordination of secondary schemes and their applications to new situations<br>• Associates symbol with events<br>• Distinguishes objects from related activity<br>• Has concept of object permanence | | | |

e. Social development

| | Yes | No | Comment |
|---|---|---|---|
| • Recognizes parents<br>• Has fear of strangers<br>• Holds arms out to be picked up<br>• Imitates others<br>• Has definite likes and dislikes<br>• Searches for dropped objects | | | |

f. Language

| | Yes | No | Comment |
|---|---|---|---|
| • Imitates sounds<br>• Laughs aloud<br>• Takes pleasure in hearing over sounds<br>• Comprehends meaning to simple words<br>• Obeys simple commands and responds to that name | | | |

g. Play

| | Yes | No | Comment |
|---|---|---|---|
| • Plays alone<br>• Plays with toys | | | |

## VI. Immunization

| Vaccine | At birth | 1 | 2 | 3 | 4 | 5 | 1st booster | 2nd booster |
|---|---|---|---|---|---|---|---|---|
| BCG | | | | | | | | |
| DPT | | | | | | | | |
| OPV | | | | | | | | |
| Measles | | | | | | | | |
| Hepatitis B | | | | | | | | |
| TT | | | | | | | | |
| MMR | | | | | | | | |
| Others | | | | | | | | |

## VII. Health Teaching

## VIII. Summary

# ASSIGNMENT–21 (A): PHYSICAL HEALTH ASSESSMENT FOR TODDLER

**I. Demographic Data**

Age: ______________________

Date of birth: ______________________

Sex: ______________________

Classification: ______________________

Head of the family: ______________________

Address: ______________________

______________________

______________________

**II. Birth History**

**Antenatal history**

Antenatal checkup: Yes/No

Immunization: Yes/No

Exposure to drug: ______________________

Viral infection: Yes/No

**Natal history**

Place of birth: hospital/home

Mode of delivery: normal/LSCS/instrumental

Gestation: Term/preterm/postmature

Delivery conducted by: Trained/untrained personnel

Condition at birth: active/asphyxiated/______________

Congenital abnormalities: Yes/No

If yes, specify ______________________

Complication if any ______________________

Birth weight ______________________

**Postnatal history**

BABY:

1. Birth injury Yes/No
2. Icterus Yes/No
3. Eye discharge Yes/No
4. Umbilical infection Yes/No

MOTHER: ______________________

Any complication ______________________

**Health History**

**Family health history**

______________________

______________________

______________________

______________________

______________________

**Past medical/surgical history**

____________________________________________________________

____________________________________________________________

____________________________________________________________

**Present health history**

____________________________________________________________

____________________________________________________________

____________________________________________________________

## III. Physical Assessment

1. **Vital signs** :Temperature ____________, Heart rate ____________, Respiration ____________
2. **Head**
   - Fontanelle :Bulged/sunken/closed/normal
   - Size :Microcephly/hydrocephalus/normal
   - Hair color :Flag sign/dry/thin/normal
   - Distribution :Equal/partial/alopecia
   - Dandruff :Present/absent
3. **Eyes**
   - Eyebrows :Absent/present
   - Eyelashes :Absent/present
   - Follicle/sty :Absent/present
   - Eyelids :Absent/present
   - Edema :Absent/present
   - Lesion :Absent/present
   - Eyeballs :Protruded/sunken/normal
4. **Conjunctiva**
   - Color :Pale/red/yellow tinged/blue tinged
   - Cornea :Transparent/smooth/moist
   - Visual acuity :Normal/myopia/hyperopia
   - Eye movement :Normal/Strabismus (squint)
   - Blurred/double vision :Absent/present
   - Polyps :Absent/present
5. **Mouth and pharynx**
   - a. Mucous membrane :Normal/red/swelling cyanosis
   - b. Breath :Normal/halitosis
   - c. Throat :Normal/sore throat/enlarged tonsils
   - d. Gum :Normal/bleeding gum/gingivitis
   - f. Tongue :Cyanotic/pale/moist/dry/coated/ulcers
   - g. Oral hygienic habits :Brushing __________ times/day
   - h. Material used :Brush/neem stick/fingers
   - i. Dentifrices :Tooth powder/toothpaste/ash/mud
6. **Neck**
   - Lymph node :Enlarged/normal
   - Thyroid gland :Normal/enlarged/midline/smooth/firm/non-tender
7. **Chest**
   - Shape :Normal/barrel shaped/pigeon chest
   - Chest movement :Symmetrical/asymmetrical
8. **Heart**
   - Position of the heart :Right/left
   - Heart sound :Normal/murmur/bruit

9. **Breasts**
   Size :Normal/abnormal-specify
   Position :Normal/abnormal
10. **Axillaries lymph nodes** :Palpable/non-palpable
11. **Abdomen**
   Skin :Rash/lesion/scars
   Umbilical
   Peristalsis :Visible/not visible
   Size :Normal/abnormal
   Bowel sound :Absent/present
12. **Genitals**
   a. Scrotal swelling or mass :Absent/present
   b. Lymph nodes :Palpable/not palpable
13. **Lower extremities**
   a. Gait :Normal/abnormal
   b. Contour :Normal/locked knee
   c. Mobility (Range of motion) :Normal/limited
14. **Integumentary system**
   a. Skin color :Normal/dark pigmented/smooth/soft/dry
   b. Temperature :Normal/cold/warm/dry
   c. Nails :Normal/blue/yellow/clubbing

## ANTHROPOMETRIC MEASUREMENT

Height/weight/HCC/CC/MAC

_______________________________________________

Diet pattern : 24 hours recall

Infants

Feeding : Breast/artificial ______________ times/day and night
Supplementary feeding ______________ times/day and night
Weaning : ______________ month

## Nutritional History

| Food items | Cooked items | Raw amount | Calorie (k cal) | Proteins (g) | Fat | Calcium (mg) | Vitamin A | Iron |
|---|---|---|---|---|---|---|---|---|
| Breakfast<br>Midmorning Lunch<br>Tea<br>Dinner | | | | | | | | |
| Total intake | | | | | | | | |
| Requirement | | | | | | | | |
| Excess/deficit | | | | | | | | |

$$\text{Degree of malnutrition} = \frac{\text{Actual weight of the child}}{\text{Expected weight}} \times 10$$

### V. Developmental Milestones: For Toddler

| Milestone | Book picture | Child's picture | Remark achieved/delayed |
|---|---|---|---|
| **A. Sensory development** | | | |
| a. Looks at picture attentively for longer period | | | |
| b. Identifies geometric forms | | | |
| c. Recalls visual images | | | |
| **B. Gross motor development** | | | |
| a. Assumes standing position without feet | | | |
| b. Walks with wide based gait | | | |
| c. Kneels without support | | | |
| d. Creeps upstairs | | | |
| e. Runs stiffly but falls | | | |
| f. Runs well | | | |
| g. Jumps with both feet in a place | | | |
| h. Rides on walker | | | |
| **C. Fine motor development** | | | |
| a. Builds a tower of cube | | | |
| b. Makes line with crayon | | | |
| c. Imitates vertical/circular stroke | | | |
| d. Unscrews lid of a jar | | | |
| e. Opens door by turning door knob | | | |
| **D. Development of self-help skills** | | | |
| a. Feeding skills | | | |
| b. Ability to use a cup | | | |
| c. Ability to use a drink | | | |
| d. Preference for finger feeding | | | |
| e. Dressing skills | | | |
| f. Removes socks and shoes | | | |
| g. Unzips garments | | | |
| h. Removes lace | | | |
| i. Toileting and grooming skills | | | |
| j. Indicates the need for toileting | | | |
| k. Bowel and bladder control | | | |
| l. Brushes teeth | | | |
| **E. Emotional and social** | | | |
| a. Tolerates separation from parents | | | |
| b. Less fearful of strangers | | | |
| c. Uses no against wishes | | | |
| d. Has great sense of mine | | | |
| e. Pulls other sense of mine | | | |
| **F. Language development** | | | |
| a. Comprehends more than can communicate | | | |
| b. Says words | | | |
| c. Shakes head to communicate no | | | |
| d. Questions the events and objectives | | | |
| e. Uses sentences | | | |
| **G. Intellectual development** | | | |
| a. Remembers objects | | | |
| b. Very curious about environment and explores the environment | | | |
| c. Actively searches the object not visible to all | | | |
| d. Searches for object in a previously known place than traces other possible places. | | | |

## VI. Immunization

| Vaccine | At birth | 1 | 2 | 3 | 4 | 5 | 1st booster | 2nd booster |
|---|---|---|---|---|---|---|---|---|
| BCG | | | | | | | | |
| DPT | | | | | | | | |
| OPV | | | | | | | | |
| Measles | | | | | | | | |
| Hepatitis B | | | | | | | | |
| TT | | | | | | | | |
| MMR | | | | | | | | |
| Others | | | | | | | | |

## VII. Health Teaching

## VIII. Summary

# ASSIGNMENT–21 (B): PHYSICAL HEALTH ASSESSMENT FOR TODDLER

## I. Demographic Data

Age: ___________________________

Date of birth: ___________________________

Sex: ___________________________

Classification: ___________________________

Head of the family: ___________________________

Address: ___________________________

___________________________

___________________________

## II. Birth History

**Antenatal history**

Antenatal checkup: Yes/No

Immunization: Yes/No

Exposure to drug: ___________________________

Viral infection: Yes/No

**Natal history**

Place of birth Hospital/home

Mode of delivery Normal/LSCS/Instrumental

Gestation Term/preterm/postmature

Delivery conducted by Trained/untrained personnel

Condition at birth Active/asphyxiated/___________

Congenital abnormalities Yes/No

If yes, specify ___________________________

Complication if any ___________________________

Birth weight ___________________________

**Postnatal history**

BABY:

1. Birth injury Yes/No
2. Icterus Yes/No
3. Eye discharge Yes/No
4. Umbilical infection Yes/No

MOTHER: ___________________________

Any complication ___________________________

## Health History

**Family health history**

___________________________

___________________________

___________________________

___________________________

**Past medical/surgical history**

___

___

___

**Present health history**

___

___

___

___

## III. Physical Assessment

1. **Vital sign** :Temperature ________, Heart rate ________, Respiration ________
2. **Head:**
   - Fontanelle :Bulged/sunken/closed/normal
   - Size :Microcephly/hydrocephalus/normal
   - Hair color :Flag sign/dry/thin/normal
   - Distribution :Equal/partial/alopecia
   - Dandruff :Present/absent
3. **Eyes**
   - Eyebrows :Absent/present
   - Eyelashes :Absent/present
   - Follicle/sty :Absent/present
   - Eyelids :Absent/present
   - Edema :Absent/present
   - Lesion :Absent/present
   - Eyeballs :Protruded/sunken/normal
4. **Conjunctiva**
   - Color :Pale/red/yellow tinged/blue tinged
   - Cornea :Transparent/smooth/moist
   - Visual acuity :Normal/myopia/hyperopia
   - Eye movement :Normal/strabismus (squint)
   - Blurred/double vision :Absent/present
   - Polyps :Absent/present
5. **Mouth and pharynx**
   - a. Mucous membrane :Normal/red/swelling cyanosis
   - b. Breath :Normal/halitosis
   - c. Throat :Normal/sore throat/enlarged tonsils
   - d. Gum :Normal/bleeding gum/gingivitis
   - f. Tongue :Cyanotic/pale/moist/dry/coated/ulcers
   - g. Oral hygienic habits :Brushing ________ times/day
   - h. Material used :Brush/neem stick/fingers
   - i. Dentifrices :Tooth powder/toothpaste/ash/mud
6. **Neck**
   - Lymph node :Enlarged/normal
   - Thyroid gland :Normal/enlarged/midline/smooth/firm/non-tender
7. **Chest**
   - Shape :Normal/barrel shaped/pigeon chest
   - Chest movement :Symmetrical/asymmetrical
8. **Heart:**
   - Position of the heart :Right/left
   - Heart sound :Normal/murmur/Bruit

9. **Breasts**
   Size :Normal/abnormal-specify
   Position :Normal/abnormal
10. **Axillaries lymph nodes** :Palpable/non-palpable
11. **Abdomen**
   Skin :Rash/lesion/scars
   Umbilical
   Peristalsis :Visible/not visible
   Size :Normal/abnormal
   Bowel sound :Absent/present
12. **Genitals**
   a. Scrotal swelling or mass :Absent/present
   b. Lymph nodes :Palpable/not palpable
13. **Lower extremities:**
   a. Gait :Normal/abnormal
   b. Contour :Normal/locked knee
   c. Mobility (Range of motion) :Normal/limited
14. **Integumentary system**
   a. Skin color :Normal/dark pigmented/ smooth/soft/dry
   b. Temperature :Normal/cold/warm/dry
   c. Nails :Normal/blue/yellow/clubbing

## ANTHROPOMETRIC MEASUREMENT

Height/weight/HCC/CC/MAC

_______________________________

Diet pattern: 24 hours recall

**Infants:**

Feeding: Breast/artificial ____________ times/day and night

Supplementary feeding ____________ times/day and night

Weaning : ____________ month

**Nutritional History:**

| Food items | Cooked items | Raw amount | Calorie (k cal) | Proteins (g) | Fat | Calcium (mg) | Vitamin A | Iron |
|---|---|---|---|---|---|---|---|---|
| Breakfast<br>Midmorning Lunch<br>Tea<br>Dinner | | | | | | | | |
| Total intake | | | | | | | | |
| Requirement | | | | | | | | |
| Excess/deficit | | | | | | | | |

$$\text{Degree of malnutrition} = \frac{\text{Actual weight of the child}}{\text{Expected weight}} \times 10$$

## V. Developmental Milestones: For Toddler

| Milestone | Book picture | Child's picture | Remark achieved/delayed |
|---|---|---|---|
| **A. Sensory development** | | | |
| a. Looks at picture attentively for longer period | | | |
| b. Identifies geometric forms | | | |
| c. Recalls visual images | | | |
| **B. Gross motor development** | | | |
| a. Assumes standing position without feet | | | |
| b. Walks with wide based gait | | | |
| c. Kneels without support | | | |
| d. Creeps upstairs | | | |
| e. Runs stiffly but falls | | | |
| f. Runs well | | | |
| g. Jumps with both feet in a place | | | |
| h. Rides on walker | | | |
| **C. Fine motor development** | | | |
| a. Builds a tower of cube | | | |
| b. Makes line with crayon | | | |
| c. Imitates vertical/circular stroke | | | |
| d. Unscrews lid of a jar | | | |
| e. Opens door by turning door knob | | | |
| **D. Development of self-help skills** | | | |
| a. Feeding skills | | | |
| b. Ability to use a cup | | | |
| c. Ability to use a drink | | | |
| d. Preference for finger feeding | | | |
| e. Dressing skills | | | |
| f. Removes socks and shoes | | | |
| g. Unzips garments | | | |
| h. Removes lace | | | |
| i. Toileting and grooming skills | | | |
| j. Indicates the need for toileting | | | |
| k. Bowel and bladder control | | | |
| l. Brushes teeth | | | |
| **E. Emotional and social** | | | |
| a. Tolerates separation from parents | | | |
| b. Less fearful of strangers | | | |
| c. Uses no against wishes | | | |
| d. Has great sense of mine | | | |
| e. Pulls other sense of mine | | | |
| **F. Language development** | | | |
| a. Comprehends more than can communicate | | | |
| b. Says words | | | |
| c. Shakes head to communicate no | | | |
| d. Questions the events and objectives | | | |
| e. Uses sentences | | | |

*Contd...*

*Contd...*

| Milestone | Book picture | Child's picture | Remark achieved/delayed |
|---|---|---|---|
| **G. Intellectual development**<br>a. Remembers objects<br>b. Very curious about environment and explores the environment<br>c. Actively searches the object not visible to all<br>d. Searches for object in a previously known place than traces other possible places | | | |

### VI. Immunization:

| Vaccine | At birth | 1 | 2 | 3 | 4 | 5 | 1st booster | 2nd booster |
|---|---|---|---|---|---|---|---|---|
| BCG | | | | | | | | |
| DPT | | | | | | | | |
| OPV | | | | | | | | |
| Measles | | | | | | | | |
| Hepatitis B | | | | | | | | |
| TT | | | | | | | | |
| MMR | | | | | | | | |
| Others | | | | | | | | |

### VII. Health Teaching

### VIII. Summary

# ASSIGNMENT–21 (C): PHYSICAL HEALTH ASSESSMENT FOR TODDLER

## I. Demographic Data:

Age: ____________________

Date of birth: ____________________

Sex: ____________________

Classification: ____________________

Head of the family: ____________________

Address: ____________________

____________________

____________________

## II. Birth History:

**Antenatal history**

| | |
|---|---|
| Antenatal checkup: | Yes/No |
| Immunization: | Yes/No |
| Exposure to drug: ____________________ | |
| Viral infection: | Yes/No |

**Natal history**

| | |
|---|---|
| Place of birth | Hospital/home |
| Mode of delivery | Normal/LSCS/instrumental |
| Gestation | Term/preterm/postmature |
| Delivery conducted by | Trained/untrained personnel |
| Condition at birth | Active/asphyxiated/ __________ |
| Congenital abnormalities | Yes/No |

If yes, specify ____________________

Complication if any ____________________

Birth weight ____________________

**Postnatal history**

BABY:

| | |
|---|---|
| 1. Birth injury | Yes/No |
| 2. Icterus | Yes/No |
| 3. Eye discharge | Yes/No |
| 4. Umbilical infection | Yes/No |

MOTHER: ____________________

Any complication ____________________

**Health History**

**Family health history**

____________________

____________________

____________________

____________________

____________________

**Past medical/surgical history**

________________________________________________

________________________________________________

________________________________________________

________________________________________________

**Present health history**

________________________________________________

________________________________________________

________________________________________________

________________________________________________

**III. Physical assessment:**

1. **Vital sign** :Temperature __________, Heart rate __________, Respiration __________
2. **Head**
   - Fontanelle :Bulged/sunken/closed/normal
   - Size :Microcephly/hydrocephalus/normal
   - Hair color :Flag sign/dry/thin/normal
   - Distribution :Equal/partial/alopecia
   - Dandruff :Present/absent
3. **Eyes**
   - Eyebrows :Absent/present
   - Eyelashes :Absent/present
   - Follicle/sty :Absent/present
   - Eyelids :Absent/present
   - Edema :Absent/present
   - Lesion :Absent/present
   - Eyeballs :Protruded/sunken/normal
4. **Conjunctiva**
   - Color :Pale/red/yellow tinged/blue tinged
   - Cornea :Transparent/smooth/moist
   - Visual acuity :Normal/myopia/hyperopia
   - Eye movement :Normal/strabismus(squint)
   - Blurred/double vision :Absent/present
   - Polyps :Absent/present
5. **Mouth and pharynx**
   - a. Mucous membrane :Normal/red/swelling cyanosis
   - b. Breath :Normal/halitosis
   - c. Throat :Normal/sore throat/enlarged tonsils
   - d. Gum :Normal/bleeding gum/gingivitis
   - f. Tongue :Cyanotic/pale/moist/dry/coated/ulcers
   - g. Oral hygienic habits :Brushing ________ times/day
   - h. Material used :Brush/neem stick/fingers
   - i. Dentifrices :Tooth powder/tooth paste/ash/mud
6. **Neck**
   - Lymph node :Enlarged/normal
   - Thyroid gland :Normal/enlarged/midline/smooth/firm/non-tender
7. **Chest**
   - Shape :Normal/barrel shaped/pigeon chest
   - Chest movement :Symmetrical/asymmetrical

8. **Heart**
   Position of the heart :Right/left
   Heart sound :Normal/murmur/Bruit
9. **Breasts**
   Size :Normal/abnormal- specify
   Position :Normal/abnormal
10. **Axillaries lymph nodes** :Palpable/non-palpable
11. **Abdomen**
   Skin :Rash/lesion/scars
   Umbilical
   Peristalsis :Visible/not visible
   Size :Normal/abnormal
   Bowel sound :Absent/present
12. **Genitals**
   a. Scrotal swelling or mass :Absent/present
   b. Lymph nodes :Palpable/not palpable
13. **Lower extremities:**
   a. Gait :Normal/abnormal
   b. Contour :Normal/locked knee
   c. Mobility (Range of motion) :Normal/limited
14. **Integumentary system**
   a. Skin color :Normal/dark pigmented/smooth/soft/dry
   b. Temperature :Normal/cold/warm/dry
   c. Nails :Normal/blue/yellow/clubbing

## ANTHROPOMETRIC MEASUREMENT

Height/weight/HCC/CC/MAC

______________________________

Diet pattern : 24 hours recall

**Infants:**

Feeding: breast/artificial ______________ times/day and night
Supplementary feeding ______________ times/day and night
Weaning: ______________ month

**Nutritional History:**

| Food items | Cooked items | Raw amount | Calorie (k cal) | Proteins (g) | Fat | Calcium (mg) | Vitamin A | Iron |
|---|---|---|---|---|---|---|---|---|
| Breakfast<br>Midmorning Lunch<br>Tea<br>Dinner | | | | | | | | |
| Total intake | | | | | | | | |
| Requirement | | | | | | | | |
| Excess/deficit | | | | | | | | |

$$\text{Degree of malnutrition} = \frac{\text{Actual weight of the child}}{\text{Expected weight}} \times 10$$

### V. Developmental Milestones: For Toddler

| Milestone | Book picture | Child's picture | Remark achieved/ delayed |
|---|---|---|---|
| **A. Sensory development** | | | |
| a. Looks at picture attentively for longer period | | | |
| b. Identifies geometric forms | | | |
| c. Recalls visual images | | | |
| **B. Gross motor development** | | | |
| a. Assumes standing position without feet | | | |
| b. Walks with wide based gait | | | |
| c. Kneels without support | | | |
| d. Creeps upstairs | | | |
| e. Runs stiffly but falls | | | |
| f. Runs well | | | |
| g. Jumps with both feet in a place | | | |
| h. Rides on walker | | | |
| **C. Fine motor development** | | | |
| a. Builds a tower of cube | | | |
| b. Makes line with crayon | | | |
| c. Imitates vertical/circular stroke | | | |
| d. Unscrews lid of a jar | | | |
| e. Opens door by turning door knob | | | |
| **D. Development of self-help skills** | | | |
| a. Feeding skills | | | |
| b. Ability to use a cup | | | |
| c. Ability to use a drink | | | |
| d. Preference for finger feeding | | | |
| e. Dressing skills | | | |
| f. Removes socks and shoes | | | |
| g. Unzips garments | | | |
| h. Removes lace | | | |
| i. Toileting and grooming skills | | | |
| j. Indicates the need for toileting | | | |
| k. Bowel and bladder control | | | |
| l. Brushes teeth | | | |
| **E. Emotional and social** | | | |
| a. Tolerates separation from parents | | | |
| b. Less fearful of strangers | | | |
| c. Uses no against wishes | | | |
| d. Has great sense of mine | | | |
| e. Pulls other sense of mine | | | |
| **F. Language development** | | | |
| a. Comprehends more than can communicate | | | |
| b. Says words | | | |
| c. Shakes head to communicate no | | | |
| d. Questions the events and objectives | | | |
| e. Uses sentences | | | |

*Contd...*

*Contd...*

| Milestone | Book picture | Child's picture | Remark achieved/delayed |
|---|---|---|---|
| **G. Intellectual development**<br>a. Remembers objects<br>b. Very curious about environment and explores the environment<br>c. Actively searches the object not visible to all<br>d. Searches for object in a previously known place than traces other possible places | | | |

### VI. Immunization

| Vaccine | At birth | 1 | 2 | 3 | 4 | 5 | 1st booster | 2nd booster |
|---|---|---|---|---|---|---|---|---|
| BCG | | | | | | | | |
| DPT | | | | | | | | |
| OPV | | | | | | | | |
| Measles | | | | | | | | |
| Hepatitis B | | | | | | | | |
| TT | | | | | | | | |
| MMR | | | | | | | | |
| Others | | | | | | | | |

### VII. Health Teaching

### VIII. Summary

# ASSIGNMENT–21 (D): PHYSICAL HEALTH ASSESSMENT FOR TODDLER

**I. Demographic Data:**

Age: ______________________

Date of birth: ______________________

Sex: ______________________

Classification: ______________________

Head of the family: ______________________

Address: ______________________

______________________

______________________

______________________

**II. Birth History:**

**Antenatal history**

| | |
|---|---|
| Antenatal checkup: | Yes/No |
| Immunization: | Yes/No |
| Exposure to drug: | ______________________ |
| Viral infection: | Yes/No |

**Natal history**

| | |
|---|---|
| Place of birth | Hospital/home |
| Mode of delivery | Normal/LSCS/instrumental |
| Gestation | Term/preterm/post-mature |
| Delivery conducted by | Trained/untrained personnel |
| Condition at birth | Active/asphyxiated/ ____________ |
| Congenital abnormalities | Yes/No |

If yes, specify ______________________

Complication if any ______________________

Birth weight ______________________

**Postnatal history**

BABY:

| | |
|---|---|
| 1. Birth injury | Yes/ No |
| 2. Icterus | Yes/No |
| 3. Eye discharge | Yes/No |
| 4. Umbilical infection | Yes/ No |

MOTHER: ______________________

Any complication ______________________

**Health History:**

**Family health history:**

______________________

______________________

______________________

______________________

______________________

**Past medical/surgical history**

______________________________________________
______________________________________________
______________________________________________
______________________________________________
______________________________________________

**Present health history**

______________________________________________
______________________________________________
______________________________________________
______________________________________________
______________________________________________
______________________________________________

## III. Physical assessment:

1. **Vital sign** :Temperature ____________, Heart rate ____________, Respiration ____________
2. **Head:**
   Fontanelle :Bulged/sunken/closed/normal
   Size :Microcephly/hydrocephalus/normal
   Hair color :Flag sign/dry/thin/normal
   Distribution :Equal/partial/alopecia
   Dandruff :Present/absent
3. **Eyes**
   Eyebrows :Absent/present
   Eyelashes :Absent/present
   Follicle/sty :Absent/present
   Eyelids
   Edema :Absent/present
   Lesion :Absent/present
   Eyeballs :Protruded/sunken/normal
4. **Conjunctiva**
   Color :Pale/red/yellow tinged/Blue tinged
   Cornea :Transparent/smooth/Moist
   Visual acuity :Normal/Myopia/Hyperopia
   Eye movement :Normal/Strabismus(squint)
   Blurred/double vision :Absent/present
   Polyps :Absent/present
5. **Mouth and pharynx**
   a. Mucous membrane :Normal/red/swelling cyanosis
   b. Breath :Normal/halitosis
   c. Throat :Normal/sore throat/enlarged tonsils
   d. Gum :Normal/bleeding gum/gingivitis
   f. Tongue :Cyanotic/pale/moist/dry/coated/ulcers
   g. Oral hygienic habits :Brushing ________ times/day
   h. Material used :Brush/neem stick/fingers
   i. Dentifrices :Tooth powder/toothpaste/ash/mud
6. **Neck**
   Lymph node :Enlarged/normal
   Thyroid gland :Normal/enlarged/mid line/smooth/firm/non-tender

7. **Chest**
   Shape :Normal/barrel shaped/pigeon chest
   Chest movement :Symmetrical/asymmetrical
8. **Heart**
   Position of the heart :Right/left
   Heart sound :Normal/murmur/Bruit
9. **Breasts**
   Size :Normal/abnormal-specify
   Position :Normal/abnormal
10. **Axillaries lymph nodes** :Palpable/non-palpable
11. **Abdomen**
    Skin :Rash/lesion/scars
    Umbilical
    Peristalsis :Visible/not visible
    Size :Normal/abnormal
    Bowel sound :Absent/present
12. **Genitals**
    a. Scrotal swelling or mass :Absent/present
    b. Lymph nodes :Palpable/not palpable
13. **Lower extremities:**
    a. Gait :Normal/abnormal
    b. Contour :Normal/locked knee
    c. Mobility :(Range of motion): normal/limited
14. **Integumentary system**
    a. Skin color :Normal/dark pigmented/smooth/soft/dry
    b. Temperature :Normal/cold/warm/dry
    c. Nails :Normal/blue/yellow/clubbing

## ANTHROPOMETRIC MEASUREMENT

Height/weight/HCC/CC/MAC

_______________________________________

Diet pattern: 24 hours recall
**Infants:**
Feeding: breast/artificial ____________ times/day and night
Supplementary feeding ________ times/day and night
Weaning: ________________ month

**Nutritional history:**

| Food items | Cooked items | Raw amount | Calorie (k cal) | Proteins (g) | Fat | Calcium (mg) | Vitamin A | Iron |
|---|---|---|---|---|---|---|---|---|
| Breakfast<br>Midmorning Lunch<br>Tea<br>Dinner | | | | | | | | |
| Total intake | | | | | | | | |
| Requirement | | | | | | | | |
| Excess/deficit | | | | | | | | |

$$\text{Degree of malnutrition} = \frac{\text{Actual weight of the child}}{\text{Expected weight}} \times 10$$

## V. Developmental Milestones: For Toddler

| Milestone | Book picture | Child's picture | Remark achieved/delayed |
|---|---|---|---|
| **A. Sensory development** | | | |
| a. Looks at picture attentively for longer period | | | |
| b. Identifies geometric forms | | | |
| c. Recalls visual images | | | |
| **B. Gross motor development** | | | |
| a. Assumes standing position without feet | | | |
| b. Walks with wide based gait | | | |
| c. Kneels without support | | | |
| d. Creeps upstairs | | | |
| e. Runs stiffly but falls | | | |
| f. Runs well | | | |
| g. Jumps with both feet in a place | | | |
| h. Rides on walker | | | |
| **C. Fine motor development** | | | |
| a. Builds a tower of cube | | | |
| b. Makes line with crayon | | | |
| c. Imitates vertical/circular stroke | | | |
| d. Unscrews lid of a jar | | | |
| e. Opens door by turning door knob | | | |
| **D. Development of self-help skills** | | | |
| a. Feeding skills | | | |
| b. Ability to use a cup | | | |
| c. Ability to use a drink | | | |
| d. Preference for finger feeding | | | |
| e. Dressing skills | | | |
| f. Removes socks and shoes | | | |
| g. Unzips garments | | | |
| h. Removes lace | | | |
| i. Toileting and grooming skills | | | |
| j. Indicates the need for toileting | | | |
| k. Bowel and bladder control | | | |
| l. Brushes teeth | | | |
| **E. Emotional and social** | | | |
| a. Tolerates separation from parents | | | |
| b. Less fearful of strangers | | | |
| c. Uses no against wishes | | | |
| d. Has great sense of mine | | | |
| e. Pulls other sense of mine | | | |
| **F. Language development** | | | |
| a. Comprehends more than can communicate | | | |
| b. Says words | | | |
| c. Shakes head to communicate no | | | |
| d. Questions the events and objectives | | | |
| e. Uses sentences | | | |
| **G. Intellectual development** | | | |
| a. Remembers objects | | | |
| b. Very curious about environment and explores the environment | | | |
| c. Actively searches the object not visible to all | | | |
| d. Searches for object in a previously known place than traces other possible places | | | |

**VI. Immunization:**

| Vaccine | At birth | 1 | 2 | 3 | 4 | 5 | 1st booster | 2nd booster |
|---|---|---|---|---|---|---|---|---|
| BCG | | | | | | | | |
| DPT | | | | | | | | |
| OPV | | | | | | | | |
| Measles | | | | | | | | |
| Hepatitis B | | | | | | | | |
| TT | | | | | | | | |
| MMR | | | | | | | | |
| Others | | | | | | | | |

**VII. Health Teaching**

**VIII. Summary**

# ASSIGNMENT–21 (E): PHYSICAL HEALTH ASSESSMENT FOR TODDLER

## I. Demographic Data

Age: ____________________

Date of birth: ____________________

Sex: ____________________

Classification: ____________________

Head of the family: ____________________

Address: ____________________

________________________________________

________________________________________

## II. Birth History

**Antenatal history**

| | |
|---|---|
| Antenatal checkup: | Yes/No |
| Immunization: | Yes/No |
| Exposure to drug: ____________________ | |
| Viral infection: | Yes/No |

**Natal history**

| | |
|---|---|
| Place of birth | Hospital/home |
| Mode of delivery | Normal/LSCS/instrumental |
| Gestation | Term/preterm/post-mature |
| Delivery conducted by | Trained/untrained personnel |
| Condition at birth | Active/asphyxiated/ ____________ |
| Congenital abnormalities | Yes/No |

If yes, specify ____________________

Complication if any ____________________

Birth weight ____________________

**Postnatal history**

BABY:

| | |
|---|---|
| 1. Birth injury | Yes/No |
| 2. Icterus | Yes/No |
| 3. Eye discharge | Yes/No |
| 4. Umbilical infection | Yes/No |

MOTHER: ____________________

Any complication ____________________

**Health History**

**Family health history:**

________________________________________

________________________________________

________________________________________

________________________________________

________________________________________

**Past medical/surgical history**

______________________________________________

______________________________________________

______________________________________________

**Present health history**

______________________________________________

______________________________________________

______________________________________________

## III. Physical Assessment

1. **Vital sign** :Temperature ________, Heart rate ________, Respiration ________
2. **Head:**
   - Fontanelle :Bulged/sunken/closed/normal
   - Size :Microcephly/hydrocephalus/normal
   - Hair color :Flag sign/dry/thin/normal
   - Distribution :Equal/partial/alopecia
   - Dandruff :Present/absent
3. **Eyes**
   - Eyebrows :Absent/present
   - Eyelashes :Absent/present
   - Follicle/sty :Absent/present
   - Eyelids
   - Edema :Absent/present
   - Lesion :Absent/present
   - Eyeballs :Protruded/sunken/normal
4. **Conjunctiva**
   - Color :Pale/red/yellow tinged/blue tinged
   - Cornea :Transparent/smooth/moist
   - Visual acuity :Normal/myopia/hyperopia
   - Eye movement :Normal/Strabismus (squint)
   - Blurred/double vision :Absent/present
   - Polyps :Absent/present
5. **Mouth and pharynx**
   - a. Mucous membrane :Normal/red/swelling cyanosis
   - b. Breath :Normal/halitosis
   - c. Throat :Normal/sore throat/enlarged tonsils
   - d. Gum :Normal/bleeding gum/gingivitis
   - f. Tongue :Cyanotic/pale/moist/dry/coated/ulcers
   - g. Oral hygienic habits :Brushing ________ times/day
   - h. Material used :Brush/neem stick/fingers
   - i. Dentifrices :Tooth powder/tooth paste/ash/ mud
6. **Neck**
   - Lymph node :Enlarged/normal
   - Thyroid gland :Normal/enlarged/mid line/smooth/firm/non-tender
7. **Chest**
   - Shape :Normal/barrel shaped/pigeon chest
   - Chest movement :Symmetrical/asymmetrical
8. **Heart**
   - Position of the heart :Right/left
   - Heart sound :Normal/murmur/Bruit

9. **Breasts**
   Size :Normal/abnormal-specify
   Position :Normal/abnormal
10. **Axillaries lymph nodes** :Palpable/non-palpable
11. **Abdomen**
   Skin :Rash/lesion/scars/
   Umbilical
   Peristalsis :Visible/not visible
   Size :Normal/abnormal
   Bowel sound :Absent/present
12. **Genitals**
   a. Scrotal swelling or mass :Absent/present
   b. Lymph nodes :Palpable/not palpable
13. **Lower extremities:**
   a. Gait :Normal/abnormal
   b. Contour :Normal/locked knee
   c. Mobility (Range of motion) :Normal/limited
14. **Integumentary system**
   a. Skin color :Normal/dark pigmented/smooth/soft/dry
   b. Temperature :Normal/cold/warm/dry
   c. Nails :Normal/blue/yellow/clubbing

## ANTHROPOMETRIC MEASUREMENT

Height/weight/HCC/CC/MAC

____________________________________

Diet pattern : 24 hours recall

**Infants**

Feeding: Breast/artificial ________________ times/day and night
Supplementary feeding ______________ times/day and night
Weaning: ____________________ month

**Nutritional History:**

| Food items | Cooked items | Raw amount | Calorie (k cals) | Proteins (g) | Fat | Calcium (mg) | Vitamin A | Iron |
|---|---|---|---|---|---|---|---|---|
| Breakfast<br>Midmorning<br>Lunch<br>Tea<br>Dinner | | | | | | | | |
| Total intake | | | | | | | | |
| Requirement | | | | | | | | |
| Excess/deficit | | | | | | | | |

$$\text{Degree of malnutrition} = \frac{\text{Actual weight of the child}}{\text{Expected weight}} \times 10$$

### V. Developmental Milestones: For Toddler

| Milestone | Book picture | Child's picture | Remark achieved/delayed |
|---|---|---|---|
| **A. Sensory development**<br>a. Looks at picture attentively for longer period<br>b. Identifies geometric forms<br>c. Recalls visual images<br>**B. Gross motor development**<br>a. Assumes standing position without feet<br>b. Walks with wide based gait<br>c. Kneels without support<br>d. Creeps upstairs<br>e. Runs stiffly but falls<br>f. Runs well<br>g. Jumps with both feet in a place<br>h. Rides on walker<br>**C. Fine motor development**<br>a. Builds a tower of cube<br>b. Makes line with crayon<br>c. Imitates vertical/circular stroke<br>d. Unscrews lid of a jar<br>e. Opens door by turning door knob<br>**D. Development of self-help skills**<br>a. Feeding skills<br>b. Ability to use a cup<br>c. Ability to use a drink<br>d. Preference for finger feeding<br>e. Dressing skills<br>f. Removes socks and shoes<br>g. Unzips garments<br>h. Removes lace<br>i. Toileting and grooming skills<br>j. Indicates the need for toileting<br>k. Bowel and bladder control<br>l. Brushes teeth<br>**E. Emotional and social**<br>a. Tolerates separation from parents<br>b. Less fearful of strangers<br>c. Uses no against wishes<br>d. Has great sense of mine<br>e. Pulls other sense of mine<br>**F. Language development**<br>a. Comprehends more than can communicate<br>b. Says words<br>c. Shakes head to communicate no<br>d. Questions the events and objectives<br>e. Uses sentences<br>**G. Intellectual development**<br>a. Remembers objects<br>b. Very curious about environment and explores the environment<br>c. Actively searches the object not visible to all<br>d. Searches for object in a previously known place than traces other possible places | | | |

**VI. Immunization:**

| Vaccine | At birth | 1 | 2 | 3 | 4 | 5 | 1st booster | 2nd booster |
|---|---|---|---|---|---|---|---|---|
| BCG | | | | | | | | |
| DPT | | | | | | | | |
| OPV | | | | | | | | |
| Measles | | | | | | | | |
| Hepatitis B | | | | | | | | |
| TT | | | | | | | | |
| MMR | | | | | | | | |
| Others | | | | | | | | |

**VII. Health Teaching**

**VIII. Summary**

# ASSIGNMENT–22 (A): PHYSICAL HEALTH FOR SCHOOL-GOING CHILDREN

**Demographic Data**

Name: ____________________

Age: ____________________

Sex: ____________________

Date of birth: ____________________

Educational status: ____________________

Head of the family: ____________________

Address: ____________________

## 1. HEALTH HISTORY

**Family health history**

**Past medical/surgical history**

**Present health history**

**Menstrual history**

- Age at menarche :
- Cycle :Regular/irregular

**Immunization**

- TAB
- Cholera
- DT
- TT
- Others

## 2. PHYSICAL EXAMINATION

a. **General appearance**
   - Body built
   - Posture
   - Behavior

b. **Vital sign**
   - Temperature
   - Pulse
   - Respiration

c. **Anthropometric assessment**
   - Height
   - Weight
   - Head circumference
   - Chest circumference

d. **Head**
   - Hair
   - Scalp

e. **Eyes**
   - Eyebrows
   - Eyelids
   - Corneal reflex

f. **Nose**
   - Size and shape
   - Discharge

g. **Mouth**
   - Lips
   - Teeth
   - Gums
   - Tongue

h. **Neck**
   - Trachea
   - Lymph node

i. **Chest**
   - Shape
   - Movement
   - Respiration rate
   - Breath sounds
   - Palpitation

**j. Abdomen**

Inspection
- Contour
- Ascites
- Visible vein
- Swelling
- Umbilicus

Palpation
- Palpable mass
- Hepatomegaly
- Splenomegaly
- Tenderness

Auscultation
- Bowel sounds

**k. Back**
- Lumbar curve
- Spinal skin appearance
- Tenderness

**l. Genitalia**

**Nutritional history:**

| Food items | Cooked items | Raw amount | Calorie (k cals) | Proteins (g) | Fat | Calcium (mg) | Vitamin A | Iron |
|---|---|---|---|---|---|---|---|---|
| Breakfast<br>Midmorning Lunch<br>Tea<br>Dinner | | | | | | | | |
| Total intake | | | | | | | | |
| Requirement | | | | | | | | |
| Excess/deficit | | | | | | | | |

$$\text{Degree of malnutrition} = \frac{\text{Actual weight of the child}}{\text{Expected weight}} \times 10$$

**Developmental Milestone: For School-going Child**

| Milestone | Book picture | Child's picture | Remark achieved/delayed |
|---|---|---|---|
| a. Dentition<br>b. Permanent teeth erupted<br>**A. Gross motor development**<br>a. Rides bicycle<br>b. Throws a ball skillfully<br>c. Uses skipping rope well<br>**B. Fine motor development**<br>a. Draws a figure<br>b. Prints fluently<br>c. Bounces a ball<br>d. Uses sharp scissors<br>**C. Development of self-help**<br>a. Eating skills<br>b. Chews without making noise and with closed mouth<br>c. Eats with finger, spoon, fork<br>d. Handles eating utensils skillfully<br>**D. Dressing and grooming skills**<br>a. Self-bath<br>i. Prefers playing in water<br>ii. Preference for clothes<br>iii. Leaves his clothes wherever they are changed<br>iv. Toileting<br>v. Able to wash self after toileting<br>**E. Language development**<br>a. Follows more than three commands given simultaneously<br>b. Responds to praise or recognition<br>c. Enjoys telling jokes<br>d. Enjoys riddles<br>**F. Emotional and social development**<br>a. Volunteers to take part in house work<br>b. Takes interest in school activities<br>c. Easy to get along with at home<br>d. Eager to please other<br>e. Exhibits consistent manner<br>**G. Intellectual development**<br>a. Questions meaning of words<br>b. Knows days of a week, months of the year<br>c. Performs arithmetical operation, memorizes multiplication table<br>Writes number in ascending order able to perform division<br>Describes objects in relation to their own aspects<br>Can read time | | | |

**Health Teaching**

______________________________

______________________________

______________________________

______________________________

______________________________

**Summary**

# ASSIGNMENT–23 (B): PHYSICAL HEALTH ASSESSMENT FOR SCHOOL-GOING CHILDREN

**Demographic Data**

Name: ____________________

Age: ____________________

Sex: ____________________

Date of birth: ____________________

Educational status: ____________________

Head of the family: ____________________

Address: ____________________

## 1. HEALTH HISTORY

**Family health history**

**Past medical/surgical history**

**Present health history**

**Menstrual history**

- Age at menarche :
- Cycle :Regular/irregular

**Immunization**
- TAB
- Cholera
- DT
- TT
- Others

## 2. PHYSICAL EXAMINATION

**a. General appearance**
- Body built
- Posture
- Behavior

**b. Vital sign**
- Temperature
- Pulse
- Respiration

**c. Anthropometric assessment**
- Height
- Weight
- Head circumference
- Chest circumference

**d. Head**
- Hair
- Scalp

**e. Eyes**
- Eyebrows
- Eyelids
- Corneal reflex

**f. Nose**
- Size and shape
- Discharge

**g. Mouth**
- Lips
- Teeth
- Gums
- Tongue

**h. Neck**
- Trachea
- Lymph node

**i. Chest**
- Shape
- Movement
- Respiration rate
- Breath sounds
- Palpitation

j. **Abdomen**

Inspection
- Contour
- Ascites
- Visible vein
- Swelling
- Umbilicus

Palpation
- Palpable mass
- Hepatomegaly
- Splenomegaly
- Tenderness

Auscultation
- Bowel sounds

k. **Back**
- Lumbar curve
- Spinal skin appearance
- Tenderness

l. **Genitalia**

________________________________________
________________________________________
________________________________________
________________________________________
________________________________________
________________________________________
________________________________________
________________________________________

**Nutritional History:**

| Food items | Cooked items | Raw amount | Calorie (k cal) | Proteins (g) | Fat | Calcium (mg) | Vitamin A | Iron |
|---|---|---|---|---|---|---|---|---|
| Breakfast<br>Midmorning<br>Lunch<br>Tea<br>Dinner | | | | | | | | |
| Total intake | | | | | | | | |
| Requirement | | | | | | | | |
| Excess/deficit | | | | | | | | |

$$\text{Degree of malnutrition} = \frac{\text{Actual weight of the child}}{\text{Expected weight}} \times 10$$

**Developmental Milestone: For School-going Child**

| Milestone | Book picture | Child's picture | Remark achieved/ delayed |
|---|---|---|---|
| a. Dentition<br>b. Permanent teeth erupted<br>**A. Gross motor development**<br>a. Rides bicycle<br>b. Throws a ball skillfully<br>c. Uses skipping rope well<br>**B. Fine motor development**<br>a. Draws a figure<br>b. Prints fluently<br>c. Bounces a ball<br>d. Uses sharp scissors<br>**C. Development of self-help**<br>a. Eating skills<br>b. Chews without making noise and with closed mouth<br>c. Eats with finger, spoon, fork<br>d. Handles eating utensils skillfully<br>**D. Dressing and grooming skills**<br>a. Self-bath<br>i. Prefers playing in water<br>ii. Preference for clothes<br>iii. Leaves his/her clothes wherever they are changed<br>iv. Toileting<br>v. Able to wash self after toileting<br>**E. Language development**<br>a. Follows more than three commands given simultaneously<br>b. Responses to praise or recognition<br>c. Enjoys telling jokes<br>d. Enjoys riddles<br>**F. Emotional and social development**<br>a. Volunteers to take part in house work<br>b. Takes interest in school activities<br>c. Easy to get along with at home<br>d. Eager to please other<br>e. Exhibits consistent manner<br>**G. Intellectual development**<br>a. Questions meaning of words<br>b. Knows days of a week, months of the year<br>c. Performs arithmetical operation<br>Memorizes multiplication table<br>Writes number in ascending order<br>Able to perform division<br>Describes objects in relation to their own aspects<br>Can read time | | | |

**Health Teaching**

_______________________________________________

_______________________________________________

_______________________________________________

**Summary**

# ASSIGNMENT–24 (C): PHYSICAL HEALTH ASSESSMENT FOR SCHOOL-GOING CHILDREN

**Demographic Data**

Name: ______________________

Age: ______________________

Sex: ______________________

Date of birth: ______________________

Educational status: ______________________

Head of the family: ______________________

Address: ______________________

## 1. HEALTH HISTORY

**Family health history**

______________________

**Past medical/surgical history**

______________________

**Present health history**

______________________

**Menstrual history**

- Age at menarche :
- Cycle :Regular/irregular

**Immunization**

- TAB
- Cholera
- DT
- TT
- Others

## 2. PHYSICAL EXAMINATION

**a. General appearance**
- Body built
- Posture
- Behavior

**b. Vital sign**
- Temperature
- Pulse
- Respiration

**c. Anthropometric assessment**
- Height
- Weight
- Head circumference
- Chest circumference

**d. Head**
- Hair
- Scalp

**e. Eyes**
- Eyebrows
- Eyelids
- Corneal reflex

**f. Nose**
- Size and shape
- Discharge

**g. Mouth**
- Lips
- Teeth
- Gums
- Tongue

**h. Neck**
- Trachea
- Lymph node

**i. Chest**
- Shape
- Movement
- Respiration rate
- Breath sounds
- Palpitation

**j. Abdomen**

Inspection
- Contour
- Ascites
- Visible vein
- Swelling
- Umbilicus

Palpation
- Palpable mass
- Hepatomegaly
- Splenomegaly
- Tenderness

Auscultation
- Bowel sounds

**k. Back**
- Lumbar curve
- Spinal skin appearance
- Tenderness

**l. Genitalia**

______________________________________________

______________________________________________

______________________________________________

**Nutritional History**

| Food items | Cooked items | Raw amount | Calorie (k cal) | Proteins (g) | Fat | Calcium (mg) | Vitamin A | Iron |
|---|---|---|---|---|---|---|---|---|
| Breakfast<br>Midmorning Lunch<br>Tea<br>Dinner | | | | | | | | |
| Total intake | | | | | | | | |
| Requirement | | | | | | | | |
| Excess/deficit | | | | | | | | |

$$\text{Degree of malnutrition} = \frac{\text{Actual weight of the child}}{\text{Expected weight}} \times 10$$

**Developmental Milestone: For School-going Child**

| Milestone | Book picture | Child's picture | Remark achieved/ delayed |
|---|---|---|---|
| a. Dentition<br>b. Permanent teeth erupted<br>**A. Gross motor development**<br>a. Rides bicycle<br>b. Throws a ball skillfully<br>c. Uses skipping rope well<br>**B. Fine motor development**<br>a. Draws a figure<br>b. Prints fluently<br>c. Bounces a ball<br>d. Uses sharp scissors | | | |

*Contd...*

*Contd...*

| Milestone | Book picture | Child's picture | Remark achieved/ delayed |
|---|---|---|---|
| **C. Development of self-help**<br>a. Eating skills<br>b. Chews without making noise and with closed mouth<br>c. Eats with finger, spoon, fork<br>d. Handles eating utensils skillfully | | | |
| **E. Language development**<br>a. Follows more than three commands given simultaneously<br>b. Responds to praise or recognition<br>c. Enjoys telling jokes<br>d. Enjoys riddles | | | |
| **F. Emotional and social development**<br>a. Volunteers to take part in house work<br>b. Takes interest in school activities<br>c. Easy to get along with at home<br>d. Eager to please other<br>e. Exhibits consistent manner | | | |
| **G. Intellectual development**<br>a. Questions meaning of words<br>b. Knows days of a week, months of the year<br>c. Performs arithmetical operation, memorizes multiplication table<br>Writes number in ascending order, able to perform division<br>Describes objects in relation to their own aspects<br>Can read time | | | |

**Health Teaching**

**Summary**

# ASSIGNMENT–22 (D): PHYSICAL HEALTH ASSESSMENT FOR SCHOOL-GOING CHILDREN

**Demographic Data**

Name: ______________________________

Age: ______________________________

Sex: ______________________________

Date of birth: ______________________________

Educational status: ______________________________

Head of the family: ______________________________

Address: ______________________________

## 1. HEALTH HISTORY

**Family health history**

**Past medical/surgical history**

**Present health history**

**Menstrual history**

- Age at menarche :
- Cycle :Regular/irregular

**Immunization**

- TAB
- Cholera
- DT
- TT
- Others

## 2. PHYSICAL EXAMINATION

a. **General appearance**
   - Body built
   - Posture
   - Behavior

b. **Vital sign**
   - Temperature
   - Pulse
   - Respiration

c. **Anthropometric assessment**
   - Height
   - Weight
   - Head circumference
   - Chest circumference

d. **Head**
   - Hair
   - Scalp

e. **Eyes**
   - Eyebrows
   - Eyelids
   - Corneal reflex

f. **Nose**
   - Size and shape
   - Discharge

g. **Mouth**
   - Lips
   - Teeth
   - Gums
   - Tongue

h. **Neck**
   - Trachea
   - Lymph node

i. **Chest**
   - Shape
   - Movement
   - Respiration rate
   - Breath sounds
   - Palpitation

j. **Abdomen**

   Inspection
   - Contour
   - Ascites
   - Visible vein

- Swelling
- Umbilicus

Palpation
- Palpable mass
- Hepatomegaly
- Splenomegaly
- Tenderness

Auscultation
- Bowel sounds

**k. Back**
- Lumbar curve
- Spinal skin appearance
- Tenderness

**l. Genitalia**

**Nutritional history:**

| Food items | Cooked items | Raw amount | Calorie (k cals) | Proteins (g) | Fat | Calcium (mg) | Vitamin A | Iron |
|---|---|---|---|---|---|---|---|---|
| Breakfast<br>Midmorning lunch<br>Tea<br>Dinner | | | | | | | | |
| Total intake | | | | | | | | |
| Requirement | | | | | | | | |
| Excess/deficit | | | | | | | | |

$$\text{Degree of malnutrition} = \frac{\text{Actual weight of the child}}{\text{Expected weight}} \times 10$$

**Developmental Milestone: For School-going Child**

| Milestone | Book picture | Child's picture | Remark achieved/ delayed |
|---|---|---|---|
| a. Dentition<br>b. Permanent teeth erupted<br>**A. Gross motor development**<br>a. Rides bicycle<br>b. Throws a ball skillfully<br>c. Uses skipping rope well<br>**B. Fine motor development**<br>a. Draws a figure<br>b. Prints fluently<br>c. Bounces a ball<br>d. Uses sharp scissors<br>**C. Development of self-help**<br>a. Eating skills<br>b. Chews without making noise and with closed mouth<br>c. Eats with finger, spoon, fork<br>d. Handles eating utensils skillfully<br>**D. Dressing and grooming skills**<br>a. Self-bath<br>i. Prefers playing in water<br>ii. Preference for clothes<br>iii. Leaves his/her clothes wherever they are changed<br>iv. Toileting<br>v. Able to wash self after toileting<br>**E. Language development**<br>a. Follows more than three commands given simultaneously<br>b. Responds to praise or recognition<br>c. Enjoys telling jokes<br>d. Enjoys riddles<br>**F. Emotional and social development**<br>a. Volunteers to take part in house work<br>b. Takes interest in school activities<br>c. Easy to get along with at home<br>d. Eager to please other<br>e. Exhibits consistent manner<br>**G. Intellectual development**<br>a. Questions meaning of words<br>b. Knows days of a week, months of the year<br>c. Performs arithmetical operation, memorizes multiplication table<br>Writes number in ascending order<br>Able to perform division<br>Describes objects in relation to their own aspects<br>Can read time | | | |

**Health Teaching**

**Summary**

# ASSIGNMENT–24 (E): PHYSICAL HEALTH ASSESSMENT FOR SCHOOL-GOING CHILDREN

**Demographic Data**

Name: ____________________

Age: ____________________

Sex: ____________________

Date of birth: ____________________

Educational status: ____________________

Head of the family: ____________________

Address: ____________________

## 1. HEALTH HISTORY

**Family health history**

**Past medical/surgical history**

**Present health history**

**Menstrual history**

- Age at menarche :
- Cycle :Regular/irregular

**Immunization**

- TAB
- Cholera
- DT
- TT
- Others

## 2. PHYSICAL EXAMINATION

**a. General appearance**
- Body built
- Posture
- Behavior

**b. Vital sign**
- Temperature
- Pulse
- Respiration

**c. Anthropometric assessment**
- Height
- Weight
- Head circumference
- Chest circumference

**d. Head**
- Hair
- Scalp

**e. Eyes**
- Eyebrows
- Eyelids
- Corneal reflex

**f. Nose**
- Size and shape
- Discharge

**g. Mouth**
- Lips
- Teeth
- Gums
- Tongue

**h. Neck**
- Trachea
- Lymph node

**i. Chest**
- Shape
- Movement
- Respiration rate

- Breath sounds
- Palpitation

**j. Abdomen**

Inspection
- Contour
- Ascites
- Visible vein
- Swelling
- Umbilicus

Palpation
- Palpable mass
- Hepatomegaly
- Splenomegaly
- Tenderness

Auscultation
- Bowel sounds

**k. Back**
- Lumbar curve
- Spinal skin appearance
- Tenderness

**l. Genitalia**

**Nutritional History**

| Food items | Cooked items | Raw amount | Calorie (k cal) | Proteins (g) | Fat | Calcium (mg) | Vitamin A | Iron |
|---|---|---|---|---|---|---|---|---|
| Breakfast<br>Midmorning<br>Lunch<br>Tea<br>Dinner | | | | | | | | |
| Total intake | | | | | | | | |
| Requirement | | | | | | | | |
| Excess/deficit | | | | | | | | |

$$\text{Degree of malnutrition} = \frac{\text{Actual weight of the child}}{\text{Expected weight}} \times 10$$

**Developmental Milestone: For School-going Child**

| Milestone | Book picture | Child's picture | Remark achieved/ delayed |
|---|---|---|---|
| a. Dentition<br>b. Permanent teeth erupted<br>**A. Gross motor development**<br>a. Rides bicycle<br>b. Throws a ball skillfully<br>c. Uses skipping rope well<br>**B. Fine motor development**<br>a. Draws a figure<br>b. Prints fluently<br>c. Bounces a ball<br>d. Uses sharp scissors<br>**C. Development of self-help**<br>a. Eating skills<br>b. Chews without making noise and with closed mouth<br>c. Eats with finger, spoon, fork<br>d. Handles eating utensils skillfully<br>**D. Dressing and grooming skills**<br>Self-bath<br>i. Prefers playing in water<br>ii. Preference for clothes<br>iii. Leaves his/her clothes wherever they are changed<br>iv. Toileting<br>v. Able to wash self after toileting<br>**E. Language development**<br>a. Follows more than three commands given simultaneously<br>b. Responds to praise or recognition<br>c. Enjoys telling jocks<br>d. Enjoys riddles<br>**F. Emotional and social development**<br>a. Volunteers to take part in house work<br>b. Takes interest in school activities<br>c. Easy to get along with at home<br>d. Eager to please other<br>e. Exhibits consistent manner<br>**G. Intellectual development**<br>a. Questions meaning words<br>b. Knows days of a week, months of the year<br>c. Performs arithmetical operation<br>Memorizes multiplication table<br>Writes number in ascending order<br>Able to perform division<br>Describes objects in relation to their own aspects<br>Can read time | | | |

## Health Teaching

___

___

___

___

**Summary**

# ASSIGNMENT–23 (A): PHYSICAL HEALTH ASSESSMENT FOR ADOLESCENCE

**Demographic Data**

Name: ____________________

Age: ____________________

Sex: ____________________

Date of birth: ____________________

Educational status: ____________________

Head of the family: ____________________

Address: ____________________

## 1. HEALTH HISTORY

**Family health history**

**Past medical/surgical history**

**Present health history**

**Menstrual history**

Age at menarche :

Cycle :Regular/irregular

**Immunization**

- TAB
- Cholera
- DT
- TT
- Others

## 2. PHYSICAL EXAMINATION

a. **General appearance**
- Body built
- Posture
- Behavior

b. **Vital sign**
- Temperature
- Pulse
- Respiration

c. **Anthropometric assessment**
- Height
- Weight
- Head circumference
- Chest circumference

d. **Head**
- Hair
- Scalp

e. **Eyes**
- Eyebrows
- Eyelids
- Corneal reflex

f. **Nose**
- Size and shape
- Discharge

g. **Mouth**
- Lips
- Teeth
- Gums
- Tongue

h. **Neck**
- Trachea
- Lymph node

i. **Chest**
- Shape
- Movement
- Respiration rate
- Breath sounds
- Palpitation

j. **Abdomen**

Inspection
- Contour
- Ascites
- Visible vein
- Swelling
- Umbilicus

Palpation
- Palpable mass
- Hepatomegaly
- Splenomegaly
- Tenderness

Auscultation
- Bowel sounds

**k. Back**
- Lumbar curve
- Spinal skin appearance
- Tenderness

**Genitalia:**

**Nutritional History:**

| Food items | Cooked items | Raw amount | Calorie (k cal) | Proteins (g) | Fat | Calcium (mg) | Vitamin A | Iron |
|---|---|---|---|---|---|---|---|---|
| Breakfast<br>Midmorning<br>Lunch<br>Tea<br>Dinner | | | | | | | | |
| Total intake | | | | | | | | |
| Requirement | | | | | | | | |
| Excess/deficit | | | | | | | | |

$$\text{Degree of malnutrition} = \frac{\text{Actual weight of the child}}{\text{Expected weight}} \times 10$$

**Developmental Milestone: For Adolescence**

| Milestone | Remark achieved/delayed |
|---|---|
| **A. Biological development**<br>a. Weight<br>b. Height<br>**B. Appearance of secondary sexual characteristics**<br>a. Has hair growth over body<br>b. Has increase in size of breast<br>**C. Assessment of cognition**<br>a. Has ability to abstract thinking<br>b. Concerned about philosophic and social problems<br>c. Has ability to view problems comprehensively<br>**D. Identity**<br>a. Preoccupied with rapid body change<br>b. Tries out various roles<br>c. Very self centered<br>d. Has rich fantasy life<br>**E. Relationship with parents**<br>a. Has strong desire to remain dependent on parents<br>b. Has major conflicts over independence and control<br>c. Has complete emotional and physical separation from parents<br>**F. Relationship with peers**<br>a. Has strong need to identify to self-image<br>b. Explores ability to attract opposite sex<br>**G. Sexuality**<br>a. Has limited outing<br>b. Has feeling of 'being in love'<br>c. Has limited intimate relationship<br>**H. Emotionality**<br>a. Has wide mood swings<br>b. Has intense day dreaming<br>c. Has feeling of inadequacy remark | |

## Health Teaching

**Summary**

# ASSIGNMENT–23 (B): PHYSICAL HEALTH ASSESSMENT FOR ADOLESCENCE

**Demographic Data**

Name: ______________________________

Age: ______________________________

Sex: ______________________________

Date of birth: ______________________________

Educational status: ______________________________

Occupation: ______________________________

Head of the family: ______________________________

Address: ______________________________

## 1. HEALTH HISTORY

**Family health history**

**Past medical/surgical history**

**Present health history**

**Menstrual history**
Age at menarche :
Cycle :Regular/irregular

**Immunization**
- TAB
- Cholera
- DT
- TT
- Others

## 2. PHYSICAL EXAMINATION

**a. General appearance**
- Body built
- Posture
- Behavior

**b. Vital sign**
- Temperature
- Pulse
- Respiration

**c. Anthropometric assessment**
- Height
- Weight
- Head circumference
- Chest circumference

**d. Head**
- Hair
- Scalp

**e. Eyes**
- Eyebrows
- Eyelids
- Corneal reflex

**f. Nose**
- Size and shape
- Discharge

**g. Mouth**
- Lips
- Teeth
- Gums
- Tongue

**h. Neck**
- Trachea
- Lymph node

**i. Chest**
- Shape
- Movement

- Respiration rate
- Breath sounds
- Palpitation

j. **Abdomen**

Inspection
- Contour
- Ascites
- Visible vein
- Swelling
- Umbilicus

Palpation
- Palpable mass
- Hepatomegaly
- Splenomegaly
- Tenderness

Auscultation
- Bowel sounds

k. **Back**
- Lumbar curve
- Spinal skin appearance
- Tenderness

**Genitalia**

______________________________________________
______________________________________________
______________________________________________
______________________________________________
______________________________________________
______________________________________________
______________________________________________

**Nutritional History**

| Food items | Cooked items | Raw amount | Calorie (k cal) | Proteins (g) | Fat | Calcium (mg) | Vitamin A | Iron |
|---|---|---|---|---|---|---|---|---|
| Breakfast<br>Midmorning<br>Lunch<br>Dinner | | | | | | | | |
| Total intake | | | | | | | | |
| Requirement | | | | | | | | |
| Excess/deficit | | | | | | | | |

$$\text{Degree of malnutrition} = \frac{\text{Actual weight of the child}}{\text{Expected weight}} \times 10$$

**Developmental Milestone: For Adolescence**

| Milestone | Remark achieved/delayed |
|---|---|
| **A. Biological development**<br>a. Weight<br>b. Height | |
| **B. Appearance of secondary sexual characteristics**<br>a. Has hair growth over body<br>b. Has increase in size of breast | |
| **C. Assessment of cognition**<br>a. Has ability to abstract thinking<br>b. Concerned about philosophic and social problems<br>c. Has ability to view problems comprehensively | |
| **D. Identity**<br>a. Preoccupied with rapid body change<br>b. Tries out of various role<br>c. Very self centered<br>d. Has rich fantasy life | |
| **E. Relationship with parents**<br>a. Has strong desire to remain dependent on parents<br>b. Has major conflicts over independence and control<br>c. Has complete emotional and physical separation from parents | |
| **F. Relationship with peers**<br>a. Has strong need to identify to self image<br>b. Explores ability to attract opposite sex | |
| **G. Sexuality**<br>a. Has limited outing<br>b. Has feeling of 'being in love'<br>c. Has limited intimate relationship | |
| **H. Emotionality**<br>a. Has wide mood swings<br>b. Has intense day dreaming<br>c. Has feeling of inadequacy remark | |

## Health Teaching

________________________________________

________________________________________

________________________________________

________________________________________

________________________________________

________________________________________

________________________________________

________________________________________

________________________________________

________________________________________

**Summary**

# ASSIGNMENT–23 (C): PHYSICAL HEALTH ASSESSMENT FOR ADOLESCENCE

**Demographic Data**

Name: ____________________

Age: ____________________

Sex: ____________________

Date of birth: ____________________

Educational status: ____________________

Occupation: ____________________

Head of the family: ____________________

Address: ____________________

## 1. HEALTH HISTORY

**Family health history**

**Past medical/surgical history**

**Present health history**

**Menstrual history**

Age at menarche :

Cycle : Regular/irregular

**Immunization**

- TAB
- Cholera
- DT
- TT
- Others

## 2. PHYSICAL EXAMINATION

a. **General appearance**
- Body built
- Posture
- Behavior

b. **Vital sign**
- Temperature
- Pulse
- Respiration

c. **Anthropometric assessment**
- Height
- Weight
- Head circumference
- Chest circumference

d. **Head**
- Hair
- Scalp

e. **Eyes**
- Eyebrows
- Eyelids
- Corneal reflex

f. **Nose**
- Size and shape
- Discharge

g. **Mouth**
- Lips
- Teeth
- Gums
- Tongue

h. **Neck**
- Trachea
- Lymph node

i. **Chest**
- Shape
- Movement
- Respiration rate
- Breath sounds
- Palpitation

j. **Abdomen**

Inspection
- Contour
- Ascites
- Visible vein

- Swelling
- Umbilicus

Palpation
- Palpable mass
- Hepatomegaly
- Splenomegaly
- Tenderness

Auscultation
- Bowel sounds

**k. Back**
- Lumbar curve
- Spinal skin appearance
- Tenderness

**Genitalia:**

**Nutritional History:**

| Food items | Cooked items | Raw amount | Calorie (k cal) | Proteins (g) | Fat | Calcium (mg) | Vitamin A | Iron |
|---|---|---|---|---|---|---|---|---|
| Breakfast<br>Midmorning<br>Lunch<br>Tea<br>Dinner | | | | | | | | |
| Total intake | | | | | | | | |
| Requirement | | | | | | | | |
| Excess/deficit | | | | | | | | |

$$\text{Degree of malnutrition} = \frac{\text{Actual weight of the child}}{\text{Expected weight}} \times 10$$

**Developmental Milestone: For Adolescence**

| Milestone | Remark achieved/delayed |
|---|---|
| **A. Biological development**<br>a. Weight<br>b. Height<br>**B. Appearance of secondary sexual characteristics**<br>a. Has hair growth over body<br>b. Has increase in size of breast<br>**C. Assessment of cognition**<br>a. Has ability to abstract thinking<br>b. Concerned about philosophic and social problems<br>c. Has ability to view problems comprehensively<br>**D. Identity**<br>a. Preoccupied with rapid body change<br>b. Tries out of various roles<br>c. Very self centered<br>d. Has rich fantasy life<br>**E. Relationship with parents**<br>a. Has strong desire to remain dependent on parents<br>b. Has major conflicts over independence and control<br>c. Has complete emotional and physical separation from parents<br>**F. Relationship with peers**<br>a. Has strong need to identify to self image<br>b. Explores ability to attract opposite sex<br>**G. Sexuality**<br>a. Has limited outing<br>b. Has feeling of 'being in love'<br>c. Has limited intimate relationship<br>**H. Emotionality**<br>a. Has wide mood swings<br>b. Has intense day dreaming<br>c. Has feeling of inadequacy remark | |

## Health Teaching

**Summary**

# ASSIGNMENT–23 (D): PHYSICAL HEALTH ASSESSMENT FOR ADOLESCENCE

**Demographic Data**

Name: ____________________

Age: ____________________

Sex: ____________________

Date of birth: ____________________

Educational status: ____________________

Occupation: ____________________

Head of the family: ____________________

Address: ____________________

## 1. HEALTH HISTORY

**Family health history**

**Past medical/surgical history**

**Present health history**

**Menstrual history**

Age at menarche :

Cycle :Regular/irregular

**Immunization**

- TAB
- Cholera
- DT
- TT
- Others

## 2. PHYSICAL EXAMINATION

a. **General appearance**
   - Body built
   - Posture
   - Behavior

b. **Vital sign**
   - Temperature
   - Pulse
   - Respiration

c. **Anthropometric assessment**
   - Height
   - Weight
   - Head circumference
   - Chest circumference

d. **Head**
   - Hair
   - Scalp

e. **Eyes**
   - Eyebrows
   - Eyelids
   - Corneal reflex

f. **Nose**
   - Size and shape
   - Discharge

g. **Mouth**
   - Lips
   - Teeth
   - Gums
   - Tongue

h. **Neck**
   - Trachea
   - Lymph node

i. **Chest**
   - Shape
   - Movement
   - Respiration rate
   - Breath sounds
   - Palpitation

j. **Abdomen**

Inspection
- Contour
- Ascites
- Visible vein
- Swelling
- Umbilicus

Palpation
- Palpable mass
- Hepatomegaly
- Splenomegaly
- Tenderness

Auscultation
- Bowel sounds

k. **Back**
- Lumbar curve
- Spinal skin appearance
- Tenderness

**Genitalia:**

**Nutritional history:**

| Food items | Cooked items | Raw amount | Calorie (k cal) | Proteins (g) | Fat | Calcium (mg) | Vitamin A | Iron |
|---|---|---|---|---|---|---|---|---|
| Breakfast<br>Midmorning<br>Lunch<br>Tea<br>Dinner | | | | | | | | |
| Total intake | | | | | | | | |
| Requirement | | | | | | | | |
| Excess/deficit | | | | | | | | |

$$\text{Degree of malnutrition} = \frac{\text{Actual weight of the child}}{\text{Expected weight}} \times 10$$

**Developmental Milestone: For Adolescence**

| Milestone | Remark achieved/delayed |
|---|---|
| **A. Biological development**<br>a. Weight<br>b. Height<br>**B. Appearance of secondary sexual characteristics**<br>a. Has hair growth over body<br>b. Has increase in size of breast<br>**C. Assessment of cognition**<br>a. Has ability to abstract thinking<br>b. Concerned about philosophic and social problems<br>c. Has ability to view problems comprehensively<br>**D. Identity**<br>a. Preoccupied with rapid body change<br>b. Tries out of various role<br>c. Very self centered<br>d. Has rich-fantasy life<br>**E. Relationship with parents**<br>a. Has strong desire to remain dependent on parents<br>b. Has major conflicts over independence and control<br>c. Has complete emotional and physical separation from parents<br>**F. Relationship with peers**<br>a. Has strong need to identify to self-image<br>b. Explores ability to attract opposite sex<br>**G. Sexuality**<br>a. Has limited outing<br>b. Has feeling of 'being in love'<br>c. Has limited intimate relationship<br>**H. Emotionality**<br>a. Has wide mood swings<br>b. Has intense day dreaming<br>c. Has feeling of inadequacy remark | |

## Health Teaching

______________________________________________

______________________________________________

______________________________________________

______________________________________________

______________________________________________

______________________________________________

______________________________________________

______________________________________________

______________________________________________

______________________________________________

______________________________________________

______________________________________________

**Summary**

# ASSIGNMENT–23 (E): PHYSICAL HEALTH ASSESSMENT FOR ADOLESCENCE

**Demographic Data**

Name: ____________________

Age: ____________________

Sex: ____________________

Date of birth: ____________________

Educational status: ____________________

Occupation: ____________________

Head of the family: ____________________

Address: ____________________

## 1. HEALTH HISTORY

**Family health history**

**Past medical/surgical history**

**Present health history**

**Menstrual history**

Age at menarche :

Cycle :Regular/irregular

**Immunization**
- TAB
- Cholera
- DT
- TT
- Others

## 2. PHYSICAL EXAMINATION

a. **General appearance**
   - Body built
   - Posture
   - Behavior

b. **Vital sign**
   - Temperature
   - Pulse
   - Respiration

c. **Anthropometric assessment**
   - Height
   - Weight
   - Head circumference
   - Chest circumference

d. **Head**
   - Hair
   - Scalp

e. **Eyes**
   - Eyebrows
   - Eyelids
   - Corneal reflex

f. **Nose**
   - Size and shape
   - Discharge

g. **Mouth**
   - Lips
   - Teeth
   - Gums
   - Tongue

h. **Neck**
   - Trachea
   - Lymph node

i. **Chest**
   - Shape
   - Movement
   - Respiration rate
   - Breath sounds
   - Palpitation

**j. Abdomen**

Inspection
- Contour
- Ascites
- Visible vein
- Swelling
- Umbilicus

Palpation
- Palpable mass
- Hepatomegaly
- Splenomegaly
- Tenderness

Auscultation
- Bowel sounds

**k. Back**
- Lumbar curve
- Spinal skin appearance
- Tenderness

**Genitalia:**

________________________________________________________________
________________________________________________________________
________________________________________________________________
________________________________________________________________
________________________________________________________________
________________________________________________________________
________________________________________________________________
________________________________________________________________

**Nutritional history:**

| Food items | Cooked items | Raw amount | Calorie (k cal) | Proteins (g) | Fat | Calcium (mg) | Vitamin A | Iron |
|---|---|---|---|---|---|---|---|---|
| Breakfast<br>Midmorning<br>Lunch<br>Tea<br>Dinner | | | | | | | | |
| Total intake | | | | | | | | |
| Requirement | | | | | | | | |
| Excess/deficit | | | | | | | | |

$$\text{Degree of malnutrition} = \frac{\text{Actual weight of the child}}{\text{Expected weight}} \times 10$$

**Developmental Milestone: For Adolescence**

| Milestone | Remark achieved/delayed |
|---|---|
| **A. Biological development**<br>a. Weight<br>b. Height<br>**B. Appearance of secondary sexual characteristics**<br>a. Has hair growth over body<br>b. Has increase in size of breast<br>**C. Assessment of cognition**<br>a. Has ability to abstract thinking<br>b. Concerned about philosophic and social problems<br>c. Has ability to view problems comprehensively<br>**D. Identity**<br>a. Preoccupied with rapid body change<br>b. Tries out of various role<br>c. Very self centered<br>d. Has rich fantasy life<br>**E. Relationship with parents**<br>a. Has strong desire to remain dependent on parents<br>b. Has major conflicts over independence and control<br>c. Has complete emotional and physical separation from parents<br>**F. Relationship with peers**<br>a. Has strong need to identify to self-image<br>b. Explores ability to attract opposite sex<br>**G. Sexuality**<br>a. Has limited outing<br>b. Has feeling of 'being in love'<br>c. Has limited intimate relationship<br>**H. Emotionality**<br>a. Has wide mood swings<br>b. Has intense day dreaming<br>c. Has feeling of inadequacy remark | |

## Health Teaching

**Summary**

# ASSIGNMENT–24 (A): PHYSICAL HEALTH ASSESSMENT FOR ADULTS

**Demographic Data**

Name: ____________________

Age: ____________________

Sex: ____________________

Date of birth: ____________________

Marital status: ____________________

Educational status: ____________________

Occupation: ____________________

Head of the family: ____________________

Address: ____________________

## 1. HEALTH HISTORY

**Family health history**

**Past medical/surgical history**

**Present health history**

**Menstrual history**

Age at menarche :

Cycle : Regular/irregular

**Immunization**

- TAB
- Cholera
- DT
- TT
- Others

## 2. PHYSICAL EXAMINATION

a. **General appearance**
   - Body built
   - Posture
   - Behavior

b. **Vital sign**
   - Temperature
   - Pulse
   - Respiration

c. **Anthropometric assessment**
   - Height
   - Weight
   - Head circumference
   - Chest circumference

d. **Head**
   - Hair
   - Scalp

e. **Eyes**
   - Eyebrows
   - Eyelids
   - Corneal reflex

f. **Nose**
   - Size and shape
   - Discharge

g. **Mouth**
   - Lips
   - Teeth
   - Gums
   - Tongue

h. **Neck**
   - Trachea
   - Lymph node

i. **Chest**
   - Shape
   - Movement
   - Respiration rate

- Breath sounds
- Palpitation

**j. Abdomen**

Inspection
- Contour
- Ascites
- Visible vein
- Swelling
- Umbilicus

Palpation
- Palpable mass
- Hepatomegaly
- Splenomegaly
- Tenderness

Auscultation
- Bowel sounds

**k. Back**
- Lumbar curve
- Spinal skin appearance
- Tenderness

**Genitalia:**

______________________________________________

______________________________________________

______________________________________________

______________________________________________

**Nutritional history:**

| Food items | Cooked items | Raw amount | Calorie (k cal) | Proteins (g) | Fat | Calcium (mg) | Vitamin A | Iron |
|---|---|---|---|---|---|---|---|---|
| Breakfast<br>Midmorning<br>Lunch<br>Tea<br>Dinner | | | | | | | | |
| Total intake | | | | | | | | |
| Requirement | | | | | | | | |
| Excess/deficit | | | | | | | | |

$$\text{Degree of malnutrition} = \frac{\text{Actual weight of the child}}{\text{Expected weight}} \times 10$$

**Health Teaching**

**Summary**

# ASSIGNMENT–24 (B): PHYSICAL HEALTH ASSESSMENT FOR ADULTS

**Demographic Data**

Name: ______________________________

Age: ______________________________

Sex: ______________________________

Date of birth: ______________________________

Marital status: ______________________________

Educational status: ______________________________

Occupation: ______________________________

Head of the family: ______________________________

Address: ______________________________

______________________________

## 1. HEALTH HISTORY

**Family health history**

______________________________

**Past medical/surgical history**

______________________________

**Present health history**

______________________________

**Menstrual history**

Age at menarche :

Cycle :Regular/irregular

**Immunization**

- TAB
- Cholera
- DT
- TT
- Others

## 2. PHYSICAL EXAMINATION

**a. General appearance**
- Body built
- Posture
- Behavior

**b. Vital sign**
- Temperature
- Pulse
- Respiration

**c. Anthropometric assessment**
- Height
- Weight
- Head circumference
- Chest circumference

**d. Head**
- Hair
- Scalp

**e. Eyes**
- Eyebrows
- Eyelids
- Corneal reflex

**f. Nose**
- Size and shape
- Discharge

**g. Mouth**
- Lips
- Teeth
- Gums
- Tongue

**h. Neck**
- Trachea
- Lymph node

**i. Chest**
- Shape
- Movement
- Respiration rate
- Breath sounds
- Palpitation

j. **Abdomen**

Inspection
- Contour
- Ascites
- Visible vein
- Swelling
- Umbilicus

Palpation
- Palpable mass
- Hepatomegaly
- Splenomegaly
- Tenderness

Auscultation
- Bowel sounds

k. **Back**
- Lumbar curve
- Spinal skin appearance
- Tenderness

**Genitalia:**

______________________________

______________________________

______________________________

______________________________

______________________________

**Nutritional history:**

| Food items | Cooked items | Raw amount | Calorie (k cal) | Proteins (g) | Fat | Calcium (mg) | Vitamin A | Iron |
|---|---|---|---|---|---|---|---|---|
| Breakfast<br>Midmorning<br>Lunch<br>Tea<br>Dinner | | | | | | | | |
| Total intake | | | | | | | | |
| Requirement | | | | | | | | |
| Excess/deficit | | | | | | | | |

$$\text{Degree of malnutrition} = \frac{\text{Actual weight of the child}}{\text{Expected weight}} \times 10$$

**Health Teaching**

______________________________

______________________________

______________________________

______________________________

______________________________

**Summary**

# ASSIGNMENT–24 (C): PHYSICAL HEALTH ASSESSMENT FOR ADULTS

**Demographic Data**

Name: ______________________

Age: ______________________

Sex: ______________________

Date of birth: ______________________

Marital status: ______________________

Educational status: ______________________

Occupation: ______________________

Head of the family: ______________________

Address: ______________________

## 1. HEALTH HISTORY

**Family health history**

______________________

**Past medical/surgical history**

______________________

**Present health history**

______________________

**Menstrual history**

Age at menarche :

Cycle :Regular/irregular

**Immunization**

- TAB
- Cholera
- DT
- TT
- Others

## 2. PHYSICAL EXAMINATION

a. **General appearance**
   - Body built
   - Posture
   - Behavior

b. **Vital sign**
   - Temperature
   - Pulse
   - Respiration

c. **Anthropometric assessment**
   - Height
   - Weight
   - Head circumference
   - Chest circumference

d. **Head**
   - Hair
   - Scalp

e. **Eyes**
   - Eyebrows
   - Eyelids
   - Corneal reflex

f. **Nose**
   - Size and shape
   - Discharge

g. **Mouth**
   - Lips
   - Teeth
   - Gums
   - Tongue

h. **Neck**
   - Trachea
   - Lymph node

i. **Chest**
   - Shape
   - Movement
   - Respiration rate
   - Breath sounds
   - Palpitation

j. **Abdomen**

Inspection
- Contour
- Ascites
- Visible vein
- Swelling
- Umbilicus

Palpation
- Palpable mass
- Hepatomegaly
- Splenomegaly
- Tenderness

Auscultation
- Bowel sounds

k. **Back**
- Lumbar curve
- Spinal skin appearance
- Tenderness

**Genitalia:**

______________________________________________________________________

______________________________________________________________________

______________________________________________________________________

______________________________________________________________________

______________________________________________________________________

**Nutritional history:**

| Food items | Cooked items | Raw amount | Calorie (k cal) | Proteins (g) | Fat | Calcium (mg) | Vitamin A | Iron |
|---|---|---|---|---|---|---|---|---|
| Breakfast<br>Midmorning<br>Lunch<br>Tea<br>Dinner | | | | | | | | |
| Total intake | | | | | | | | |
| Requirement | | | | | | | | |
| Excess/deficit | | | | | | | | |

$$\text{Degree of malnutrition} = \frac{\text{Actual weight of the child}}{\text{Expected weight}} \times 10$$

**Health Teaching**

______________________________________________________________________

______________________________________________________________________

______________________________________________________________________

______________________________________________________________________

______________________________________________________________________

______________________________________________________________________

**Summary**

# ASSIGNMENT–24 (D): PHYSICAL HEALTH ASSESSMENT FOR ADULTS

**Demographic Data**

Name: ______________________

Age: ______________________

Sex: ______________________

Date of birth: ______________________

Marital status: ______________________

Educational status: ______________________

Occupation: ______________________

Head of the family: ______________________

Address: ______________________

## 1. HEALTH HISTORY

**Family health history**

**Past medical/surgical history**

**Present health history**

**Menstrual history**

Age at menarche :

Cycle :Regular/irregular

Age at menopause :

Menopausal symptom :Yes/No

**Immunization**

- TAB
- Cholera
- DT
- TT
- Others

## 2. PHYSICAL EXAMINATION

**a. General appearance**
- Body built
- Posture
- Behavior

**b. Vital sign**
- Temperature
- Pulse
- Respiration

**c. Anthropometric assessment**
- Height
- Weight
- Head circumference
- Chest circumference

**d. Head**
- Hair
- Scalp

**e. Eyes**
- Eyebrows
- Eyelids
- Corneal reflex

**f. Nose**
- Size and shape
- Discharge

**g. Mouth**
- Lips
- Teeth
- Gums
- Tongue

**h. Neck**
- Trachea
- Lymph node

**i. Chest**
- Shape
- Movement
- Respiration rate
- Breath sounds
- Palpitation

**j. Abdomen**

Inspection

- Contour
- Ascites
- Visible vein
- Swelling
- Umbilicus

Palpation
- Palpable mass
- Hepatomegaly
- Splenomegaly
- Tenderness

Auscultation
- Bowel sounds

**k. Back**
- Lumbar curve
- Spinal skin appearance
- Tenderness

**Genitalia:**

______________________________________________

______________________________________________

______________________________________________

______________________________________________

______________________________________________

**Nutritional History:**

| Food items | Cooked items | Raw amount | Calorie (k cal) | Proteins (g) | Fat | Calcium (mg) | Vitamin A | Iron |
|---|---|---|---|---|---|---|---|---|
| Breakfast<br>Midmorning<br>Lunch<br>Tea<br>Dinner | | | | | | | | |
| Total intake | | | | | | | | |
| Requirement | | | | | | | | |
| Excess/deficit | | | | | | | | |

$$\text{Degree of malnutrition} = \frac{\text{Actual weight of the child}}{\text{Expected weight}} \times 10$$

**Health Teaching**

______________________________________________

______________________________________________

______________________________________________

______________________________________________

______________________________________________

______________________________________________

______________________________________________

______________________________________________

**Summary**

# ASSIGNMENT–24 (E): PHYSICAL HEALTH ASSESSMENT FOR ADULTS

**Demographic Data**

Name: ____________________

Age: ____________________

Sex: ____________________

Date of birth: ____________________

Marital status: ____________________

Educational status: ____________________

Occupation: ____________________

Head of the family: ____________________

Address: ____________________

## 1. HEALTH HISTORY

**Family health history**

**Past medical/surgical history**

**Present health history**

**Menstrual history**

Age at menarche :

Cycle :Regular/irregular

Age at menopause :

Menopausal symptom :Yes/No

**Immunization**

- TAB
- Cholera
- DT
- TT
- Others

## 2. PHYSICAL EXAMINATION

**a. General appearance**
  - Body built
  - Posture
  - Behavior

**b. Vital sign**
  - Temperature
  - Pulse
  - Respiration

**c. Anthropometric assessment**
  - Height
  - Weight
  - Head circumference
  - Chest circumference

**d. Head**
  - Hair
  - Scalp

**e. Eyes**
  - Eyebrows
  - Eyelids
  - Corneal reflex

**f. Nose**
  - Size and shape
  - Discharge

**g. Mouth**
  - Lips
  - Teeth
  - Gums
  - Tongue

**h. Neck**
  - Trachea
  - Lymph node

**i. Chest**
  - Shape
  - Movement
  - Respiration rate
  - Breath sounds
  - Palpitation

j. **Abdomen**
Inspection
- Contour
- Ascites
- Visible vein
- Swelling
- Umbilicus

Palpation
- Palpable mass
- Hepatomegaly
- Splenomegaly
- Tenderness

Auscultation
- Bowel sounds

k. **Back**
- Lumbar curve
- Spinal skin appearance
- Tenderness

**Genitalia**

________________________________________
________________________________________
________________________________________
________________________________________

**Nutritional History:**

| Food items | Cooked items | Raw amount | Calorie (k cal) | Proteins (g) | Fat | Calcium (mg) | Vitamin A | Iron |
|---|---|---|---|---|---|---|---|---|
| Breakfast<br>Midmorning<br>Lunch<br>Tea<br>Dinner | | | | | | | | |
| Total intake | | | | | | | | |
| Requirement | | | | | | | | |
| Excess/deficit | | | | | | | | |

$$\text{Degree of malnutrition} = \frac{\text{Actual weight of the child}}{\text{Expected weight}} \times 10$$

**Health Teaching**

________________________________________
________________________________________
________________________________________
________________________________________
________________________________________
________________________________________

**Summary**

# ASSIGNMENT–25 (A): PHYSICAL HEALTH ASSESSMENT FOR ANTENATAL/POSTNATAL MOTHER

**Demographic Data**

Name: ____________________

Age: ____________________

Religion: ____________________

Education: ____________________

Occupation: ____________________

Classification: ____________________

Address: ____________________

Hospital no: ____________________

Husband's name: ____________________

Age: ____________________

Occupation: ____________________

**Health History**

a. Family health history
Bronchial asthma/epilepsy/HT/IHD/Communicable disease _ specify/Others ____________________

b. Personal health history
Habits: chewing/using snuff/others
Dietary habits – veg/non-veg/any restriction
Bathing: everyday/alternate day/weekly
Prefers: Hot/cold water
Bowel and bladder habits: Normal: Yes/no/regular/irregular
Allergic to: __________ specify
Others ____________________

c. Past and present medical history, if any, give the details.

d. Obstetrical history

Obstetrical score: G-P-L-A-SB-ND

Age at menarche:

Menstrual history:

Age at marriage:

Consanguineous:

LMP: EDD

Weeks of gestation:

Immunization: TT: 1st ______________ 2nd ______________

High-risk factors ________________________________________

________________________________________

________________________________________

**Mother**

| Sl. No. | Year | Duration of labor | Mode of delivery | | | Place | | By whom specify | | | | |
|---|---|---|---|---|---|---|---|---|---|---|---|---|
| | | | Normal | Instrumental | CS | Home | Hospital | Dr | Nurse | ANM | Trained dai | Untrained dai |
| | | | | | | | | | | | | |

Placental weight ________________________________________

________________________________________

Postnatal complication, if any ________________________________________

________________________________________

________________________________________

| Sl. No. | Alive birth | Stillbirth | Alive now | Condition at birth | If dead, cause |
|---|---|---|---|---|---|
| | | | | | |
| | | | | | |

## Newborn

Cried at birth: yes/no

Birth injury: yes/no

Birth weight:

APGAR score:

________________________________________

________________________________________

________________________________________

________________________________________

**Physical Assessment**

| Area of assessment | Antenatal | | | Postnatal | | |
|---|---|---|---|---|---|---|
| | Normal | Abnormal | Description | Normal | | Description |
| | | | | Yes | No | |
| • Eyes<br>• Mouth<br>• Heart<br>• Lungs<br>• Breast<br>• Nipple cracked inverted<br>• Vaginal discharge<br>• Lochia<br>• Episiotomy<br>• Urine—albumin, sugar<br>• Bowel movements<br>• Extremities | | | | | | |

**Abdomen**

Shape :Fundal height
Size :Uterus–soft/contracted/not contracted
Striae :
Palpation :
Fundal :Height of the fundus
Lie
Presentation
Pelvic :Engagement
Presenting part

**Vital signs**

- Temperature
- Pulse
- Respiration
- Blood pressure
- Anthropometric measurement
- Height
- Weight.

**Nutritional Assessment (24 hours recall)**

| Food items | Cooked items | Raw amount | Calorie (k cal) | Proteins (g) | Fat | Calcium (mg) | Vitamin A | Iron |
|---|---|---|---|---|---|---|---|---|
| Breakfast<br>Midmorning<br>Lunch<br>Tea<br>Dinner | | | | | | | | |
| Total intake | | | | | | | | |
| Requirement | | | | | | | | |
| Excess/deficit | | | | | | | | |

**Antenatal**

- Preparation for delivery: prepared/unprepared
- Preference of delivery at home/hospital
- Distance from home to hospital
- Plan to meet any medical/obstetrical emergency
- Attitudes, beliefs
  - Antenatal care
  - Delivery
  - Postpartum care
  - Newborn care
  - Family planning

**Family planning practice**

- Permanent/temporary methods
- Tubectomy
- Vasectomy
- Condom
- Copper T
- Pills

  If not adopted, reason ______________________________

  ______________________________

  ______________________________

# ASSIGNMENT–25 (B): PHYSICAL HEALTH ASSESSMENT FOR ANTENATAL/POSTNATAL MOTHER

**Demographic Data**

Name: ____________________

Age: ____________________

Religion: ____________________

Education: ____________________

Occupation: ____________________

Classification: ____________________

Address: ____________________

Hospital No: ____________________

Husband's name: ____________________

Age: ____________________

Occupation: ____________________

**Health History**

a. Family health history
   Bronchial asthma/epilepsy/HT/IHD/Communicable disease _ specify/Others ____________________

b. Personal health history
   Habits: chewing/using snuff/others
   Dietary habits – veg/non-veg/any restriction
   Bathing: Everyday/alternate day/weekly
   Prefers: Hot/cold water
   Bowel and bladder habits: Normal: Yes/no/regular/irregular
   Allergic to: ____________ specify
   Others ____________________

c. Past and present medical history, if any, give the details

d. Obstetrical history
   Obstetrical score: G-P-L-A-SB-ND
   Age at menarche:
   Menstrual history:
   Age at marriage:

Consanguineous:
LMP: EDD
Weeks of gestation:
Immunization: TT: 1st ____________ 2nd ____________
High-risk Factors ________________________________________

**Mother**

| Sl. No. | Year | Duration of labor | Mode of delivery | | | Place | | By whom specify | | | | |
|---|---|---|---|---|---|---|---|---|---|---|---|---|
| | | | Normal | Instrumental | CS | Home | Hospital | Dr | Nurse | ANM | Trained dai | Untrained dai |
| | | | | | | | | | | | | |

Placental weight ________________________________________

Postnatal complication, if any ________________________________

| Sl. No. | Alive birth | Stillbirth | Alive now | Condition at birth | If dead, cause |
|---|---|---|---|---|---|
| | | | | | |
| | | | | | |
| | | | | | |

## Newborn

Cried at birth: Yes/no
Birth-injury: Yes/no
Birth weight:
APGAR score:

**Physical Assessment**

| Area of assessment | Antenatal | | | Postnatal | | |
|---|---|---|---|---|---|---|
| | Normal | Abnormal | Description | Normal | | Description |
| | | | | Yes | No | |
| • Eyes<br>• Mouth<br>• Heart<br>• Lungs<br>• Breast<br>• Nipple cracked inverted<br>• Vaginal discharge<br>• Lochia<br>• Episiotomy<br>• Urine – Albumin, sugar<br>• Bowel movements<br>• Extremities | | | | | | |

**Abdomen**

Shape :Fundal height
Size :Uterus—soft/contracted/not contracted
Striae :
Palpation :
Fundal :Height of the fundus
Lie
Presentation
Pelvic :Engagement
Presenting part

**Vital signs:**

- Temperature
- Pulse
- Respiration
- Blood pressure
- Anthropometric measurement
- Height
- Weight.

**Nutritional assessment (24 hours recall)**

| Food items | Cooked items | Raw amount | Calorie (k cal) | Proteins (g) | Fat | Calcium (mg) | Vitamin A | Iron |
|---|---|---|---|---|---|---|---|---|
| Breakfast<br>Midmorning<br>Lunch<br>Tea<br>Dinner | | | | | | | | |
| Total intake | | | | | | | | |
| Requirement | | | | | | | | |
| Excess/deficit | | | | | | | | |

**Antenatal**

- Preparation for delivery: prepared/unprepared
- Preference of delivery at home/hospital
- Distance from home to hospital
- Plan to meet any medical/obstetrical emergency
- Attitudes, beliefs:
  - Antenatal care
  - Delivery
  - Post-partum care
  - Newborn care
  - Family planning.

**Family planning practice**

- Permanent/temporary methods
- Tubectomy
- Vasectomy
- Condom
- Copper T
- Pills.

  If not adopted, reason ________________________________________
  ________________________________________
  ________________________________________

# ASSIGNMENT–25 (C): PHYSICAL HEALTH ASSESSMENT FOR ANTENATAL/POSTNATAL MOTHER

**Demographic Data**

Name: ____________________

Age: ____________________

Religion: ____________________

Education: ____________________

Occupation: ____________________

Classification: ____________________

Address: ____________________

Hospital No: ____________________

Husband's name: ____________________

Age: ____________________

Occupation: ____________________

**Health History**

a. Family health history
Bronchial asthma/epilepsy/HT/IHD/Communicable disease _ specify/Others ____________________
____________________
____________________

b. Personal health history
Habits: Chewing/using snuff/others
Dietary habits – veg/non-veg/any restriction
Bathing: Everyday/alternate day/weekly
Prefers: Hot/cold water
Bowel and bladder habits: Normal: Yes/no/regular/irregular
Allergic to: ____________ specify
Others ____________________
____________________
____________________

c. Past and present medical history, if any, give the details
____________________
____________________
____________________
____________________

d. Obstetrical history
Obstetrical score: G-P-L-A-SB-ND
Age at menarche:
Menstrual history:
Age at marriage:
Consanguineous:
LMP: EDD
Weeks of gestation:

Immunization: TT: 1st __________ 2nd __________

High-risk Factors ______________________________

## Mother

| Sl. No. | Year | Duration of labor | Mode of delivery | | | Place | | By whom specify | | | | |
|---|---|---|---|---|---|---|---|---|---|---|---|---|
| | | | Normal | Instrumental | CS | Home | Hospital | Dr | Nurse | ANM | Trained dai | Untrained dai |
| | | | | | | | | | | | | |

Placental weight ______________________________

Postnatal complication, if any ______________________________

| Sl. No. | Alive birth | Stillbirth | Alive now | Condition at birth | If dead, cause |
|---|---|---|---|---|---|
| | | | | | |
| | | | | | |

## Newborn

Cried at birth: yes/no
Birth injury: yes/no
Birth weight:
APGAR score:

**Physical Assessment**

| Area of assessment | Antenatal | | | Postnatal | | |
|---|---|---|---|---|---|---|
| | Normal | Abnormal | Description | Normal | | Description |
| | | | | Yes | No | |
| • Eyes<br>• Mouth<br>• Heart<br>• Lungs<br>• Breast<br>• Nipple cracked inverted<br>• Vaginal discharge<br>• Lochia<br>• Episiotomy<br>• Urine – Albumin, sugar<br>• Bowel movements<br>• Extremities | | | | | | |

**Abdomen**

Shape :Fundal height
Size :Uterus – soft/contracted/not contracted
Striae :
Palpation :
Fundal :Height of the fundus
Lie
Presentation
Pelvic :Engagement
Presenting part

**Vital signs**

- Temperature
- Pulse
- Respiration
- Blood pressure
- Anthropometric measurement
- Height
- Weight

**Nutritional Assessment (24 hours recall)**

| Food items | Cooked items | Raw amount | Calorie (k cal) | Proteins (g) | Fat | Calcium (mg) | Vitamin A | Iron |
|---|---|---|---|---|---|---|---|---|
| Breakfast<br>Midmorning<br>Lunch<br>Tea<br>Dinner | | | | | | | | |
| Total intake | | | | | | | | |
| Requirement | | | | | | | | |
| Excess/deficit | | | | | | | | |

**Antenatal:**

- Preparation for delivery: Prepared/unprepared
- Preference of delivery at home/hospital
- Distance from home to hospital
- Plan to meet any medical/obstetrical emergency
- Attitudes, beliefs:
  - Antenatal care
  - Delivery
  - Postpartum care
  - Newborn care
  - Family planning.

**Family planning practice**

- Permanent/temporary methods
- Tubectomy
- Vasectomy
- Condom
- Copper T
- Pills.

If not adopted, reason ______________________________

______________________________

______________________________

# ASSIGNMENT–25 (D): PHYSICAL HEALTH ASSESSMENT FOR ANTENATAL/POSTNATAL MOTHER

**Demographic Data**

Name: ____________________

Age: ____________________

Religion: ____________________

Education: ____________________

Occupation: ____________________

Classification: ____________________

Address: ____________________

Hospital No: ____________________

Husband's name: ____________________

Age: ____________________

Occupation: ____________________

**Health History**

a. Family health history
   Bronchial asthma/epilepsy/HT/IHD/Communicable disease _ specify/Others ____________________

b. Personal health history

   Habits: Chewing/using snuff/others ____________________

   Dietary habits – veg/non-veg/any restriction ____________________

   Bathing: Everyday/alternate day/weekly ____________________

   Prefers: Hot/cold water ____________________

   Bowel and bladder habits: Normal: Yes/no/regular/irregular ____________________

   Allergic to: ____________ specify ____________________

   Others ____________________

c. Past and present medical history, if any, give the details.

d. Obstetrical history

Obstetrical score: G-P-L-A-SB-ND

Age at menarche:

Menstrual history:

Age at marriage:

Consanguineous:

LMP: EDD

Weeks of gestation:

Immunization: TT: 1st ______________ 2nd ______________

High-risk Factors ________________________________________

________________________________________

________________________________________

________________________________________

**MOTHER**

| Sl. No. | Year | Duration of labor | Mode of delivery | | | Place | | By whom specify | | | | |
|---|---|---|---|---|---|---|---|---|---|---|---|---|
| | | | Normal | Instrumental | CS | Home | Hospital | Dr. | Nurse | ANM | Trained dai | Untrained dai |
| | | | | | | | | | | | | |

Placental weight ________________________________________

________________________________________

Postnatal complication, if any ________________________________________

________________________________________

________________________________________

| Sl. No. | Alive birth | Stillbirth | Alive now | Condition at birth | If dead, cause |
|---|---|---|---|---|---|
| | | | | | |
| | | | | | |

## Newborn

Cried at birth: yes/no ________________________________________

Birth injury: yes/no ________________________________________

Birth weight: ________________________________________

APGAR score: ________________________________________

________________________________________

________________________________________

**Physical Assessment**

| Area of assessment | Antenatal | | | Postnatal | | |
|---|---|---|---|---|---|---|
| | Normal | Abnormal | Description | Normal | | Description |
| | | | | Yes | No | |
| • Eyes<br>• Mouth<br>• Heart<br>• Lungs<br>• Breast<br>• Nipple cracked Inverted<br>• Vaginal discharge<br>• Lochia<br>• Episiotomy<br>• Urine – Albumin, sugar<br>• Bowel movements<br>• Extremities | | | | | | |

**Abdomen**

Shape :Fundal height
Size :Uterus soft/contracted/not contracted
Striae :
Palpation :
Fundal :Height of the fundus
Lie
Presentation
Pelvic :Engagement
Presenting part

**Vital signs**

- Temperature
- Pulse
- Respiration
- Blood pressure
- Anthropometric measurement
- Height
- Weight

**Nutritional Assessment ( 24 hrs. recall )**

| Food items | Cooked items | Raw amount | Calorie (k cal) | Proteins (g) | Fat | Calcium (mg) | Vitamin A | Iron |
|---|---|---|---|---|---|---|---|---|
| Breakfast<br>Midmorning<br>Lunch<br>Tea<br>Dinner | | | | | | | | |
| Total intake | | | | | | | | |
| Requirement | | | | | | | | |
| Excess/deficit | | | | | | | | |

**Antenatal**

- Preparation for delivery: prepared/unprepared
- Preference of delivery at home/hospital

- Distance from home to hospital
- Plan to meet any medical/obstetrical emergency
- Attitudes, beliefs:
  - Antenatal care
  - Delivery
  - Postpartum care
  - Newborn care
  - Family planning

**Family planning practice**

- Permanent/temporary methods
- Tubectomy
- Vasectomy
- Condom
- Copper T
- Pills.

If not adopted, reason ___________________________________________
___________________________________________
___________________________________________
___________________________________________

# ASSIGNMENT–25 (E): PHYSICAL HEALTH ASSESSMENT FOR ANTENATAL/POSTNATAL MOTHER

**Demographic Data**

Name: ______________________________

Age: ______________________________

Religion: ______________________________

Education: ______________________________

Occupation: ______________________________

Classification: ______________________________

Address: ______________________________

Hospital No: ______________________________

Husband's name: ______________________________

Age: ______________________________

Occupation: ______________________________

**Health History**

a. Family health history
   Bronchial asthma/epilepsy/HT/IHD/Communicable disease _ specify/Others ______________________________

b. Personal health history
   Habits : chewing/using snuff/others
   Dietary habits – veg/non veg/any restriction
   Bathing : everyday/alternate day/weekly
   Prefers : Hot/cold water
   Bowel and bladder habits : Normal : Yes/no/regular/irregular
   Allergic to : ______________ specify
   Others ______________________________

c. Past and Present medical history if any, give the details

d. Obstetrical history
Obstetrical score: G-P-L-A-SB-ND
Age at menarche:
Menstrual history:
Age at marriage:
Consanguineous:
LMP: EDD
Weeks of gestation:
Immunization: TT: 1st ____________ 2nd ____________
High Risk Factors ____________________________________________
____________________________________________
____________________________________________
____________________________________________

**MOTHER**

| Sl. No. | Year | Duration of labour | Mode of delivery | | | Place | | By whom specify | | | | |
|---|---|---|---|---|---|---|---|---|---|---|---|---|
| | | | Normal | Instrumental | CS | Home | Hospital | Dr. | Nurse | ANM | Trained dai | Untrained dai |
| | | | | | | | | | | | | |

Placental weight ____________________________________________
____________________________________________

Postnatal complication, if any ____________________________________________
____________________________________________
____________________________________________

| Sl. No. | Alive birth | Stillbirth | Alive now | Condition at birth | If dead, cause |
|---|---|---|---|---|---|
| | | | | | |
| | | | | | |

## Newborn

Cried at birth: yes/no
Birth injury: yes/no
Birth weight:
APGAR score:
____________________________________________
____________________________________________
____________________________________________
____________________________________________
____________________________________________
____________________________________________

**Physical Assessment**

| Area of assessment | Antenatal | | | Postnatal | | |
|---|---|---|---|---|---|---|
| | Normal | Abnormal | Description | Normal | | Description |
| | | | | Yes | No | |
| • Eyes<br>• Mouth<br>• Heart<br>• Lungs<br>• Breast<br>• Nipple cracked Inverted<br>• Vaginal discharge<br>• Lochia<br>• Episiotomy<br>• Urine – Albumin, sugar<br>• Bowel movements<br>• Extremities | | | | | | |

**Abdomen**

Shape :Fundal height
Size :Uterus—soft/contracted/not contracted
Striae :
Palpation :
Fundal :Height of the fundus
Lie
Presentation
Pelvic :Engagement
Presenting part.

**Vital signs**

- Temperature
- Pulse
- Respiration
- Blood pressure
- Anthropometric measurement
- Height
- Weight.

**Nutritional Assessment (24 hours recall)**

| Food items | Cooked items | Raw amount | Calorie (k cal) | Proteins (g) | Fat | Calcium (mg) | Vitamin A | Iron |
|---|---|---|---|---|---|---|---|---|
| Breakfast<br>Midmorning lunch<br>Tea<br>Dinner | | | | | | | | |
| Total intake | | | | | | | | |
| Requirement | | | | | | | | |
| Excess/deficit | | | | | | | | |

**Antenatal:**

- Preparation for delivery: prepared/unprepared
- Preference of delivery at home/hospital

- Distance from home to hospital
- Plan to meet any medical/obstetrical emergency
- Attitudes, beliefs
  - Antenatal care
  - Delivery
  - Postpartum care
  - Newborn care
  - Family planning.

**Family planning practice**

- Permanent/temporary methods
- Tubectomy
- Vasectomy
- Condom
- Copper T
- Pills.

If not adopted, reason ____________________________________________

____________________________________________

____________________________________________

# 8. NATIONAL HEALTH POLICY

## INTRODUCTION

Policy is a system, which provides the logical framework and rationality of decision making for the achievement of intended objectives. It is statement that guides and provides discretion within limited boundaries. Policy sets priorities and guides resources.

The minister of health and family welfare, Govt. of India, evolved an NHP in 1983 keeping in view the national commitment to attain the goal of health for all. Since then, there has been significant changes in the determinant factors relating to the health sector, necessitating revision of the policy and a new NHP-2002 evolved.

## OBJECTIVES

To achieve an acceptable standard of good health amongst the general population of the country.

To increase access to the decentralized public health system by establishing new infrastructure in deficient areas and by upgrading the infrastructure in the existing institution.

To ensuring a more equitable access to health services across the social and geographical expanse of the country.

To increase the aggregate public health investment through a substantially increased contribution by the central Govt.

To strengthen the capacity of the public health administration of the state level to render effective services delivery.

To enhance the contribution of the private sector in providing health services for the population group, which can afford to pay for services.

To rationalize use of drugs within the allopathic systems.

To increase access to tried and tested systems of traditional medicine.

### *Goals Set to be Achieved*

2005: Eradicate poliomyelitis and yaws:

Eliminate leprosy:

Establish an integrated system of surveillance

National health accounts and health statistics

Increase state sector health spending from 5.5 to 7 percent of the budget.

2007: Achieve zero level growth of HIV/AIDS

2010:

Eliminate kala-azar:

Reduce mortality by 50 percent on account of TB, malaria and other vector and water-borne diseases

Reduce prevalence of blindness to 0.5 percent

Reduce IMR to 30/1000 and MMR to 1/1000

Increase utilization of public health facilities from current level of less than 20 percent to more than 75 percent
Increase health expenditure by Govt from the existing 0.9 percent to 2 percent of GDP
Increase share of central grants to constitute at least 25 percent of total health spending
Further increase of state sector health spending to 8 percent
2015: Eliminate lymphatic filariasis.

## POLICY PRESCRIPTION

1. **Financial resources:** To increase health sector expenditure to 6 percent of GDP, with 2 percent of GDP being contributed as public health investment, by the year 2010.
   State Govt, expected to increase health contribution about 7 percent of the budget by 2005 and 8 percent of the budget by 2010.
   Central Govt contribution to public health would rise to 25 percent from the existing 15 percent by 2010.
2. **Equity:** NHP – 2002, set out an increased allocation 55 percent of the total public health investment for primary health sector; the secondary and tertiary health sector being targeted for 35 percent and 10 percent respectively.
3. **Delivery of national public health program:** It is done through horizontal manner. It means giving responsibility to state Govt for scientific designing of public health projects through village and Dist health administration, depending on the local needs. Policy ensures the provisioning of financial resources, in addition to technical support, monitoring and evaluation NHP at the national level by the center.
4. **The state of public health infrastructure:** It means strengthening public health infrastructure. It is by creation of a decentralized health system, will ensure a more effective supervision of the public health personnel through community monitoring, than has been achieved through the regular administration line of controls. Provision of essential resources and drugs to strengthen the primary health structure for attaining the improved public health outcomes on an equitable basis.
5. **Extending public health services:** It includes private and Indian systems of medicine and homeopathy. The number of medical, paramedical and practitioners of other system of medicine permitted, after adequate training. Stressed on two rural posting before the awarding of the graduate degree.
6. **Role of local self-Govt institutions:** Great emphasis upon the implementation of public health program through local self-Govt institutions. The policy urges all state Govt to consider decentralizing the implementation of the programs by transferring power to such institutions.
7. **Norms for health care professionals:** Minimal statutory norms with constant reviewing for the deployment of doctors and nurses in medical institutions need to be introduced urgently under the provision of the IMC Act and INC Act, respectively.
8. **Education of health care professionals:** The setting up of a new medical grants commission for funding new Govt. medical and dental colleges in different parts of the country and also fund for the upgradation of the infrastructure of the existing colleges, to improve standard of medical education. Need-based and skill-oriented syllabus, CME, UG curriculum need to concern for geriatric disorder, forensic medicine, radiology, medical research.
9. **Need for specialists in public health and family welfare:** To raise proportion of PG seats in these disciplines in medical training to reach a stage, where-in one-fourth of the seats are earmarked for these disciplines. Specialization in public health may be encouraged for both medical doctors and non-medical graduates from the allied fields like public health engineering, microbiology and other natural sciences.
10. **Nursing personnel:** Need for an improvement in the ratio of nurses and doctors/beds in Govt. and private sector. Need for establishing training causes for superspecialty nurses required for tertiary care institutions.

11. **Use of generic drugs and vaccine:** It emphasizes on a limited number of essential drugs of a generic nature, need to be used both public and private domain. The list of essential drugs would, no doubt, have to be reviewed periodically. The production and sale of irrational combinations of drugs would be prohibited through the drug standards.
12. **Urban health:** Setting up of an organized urban primary health care (PHC) structure, which is a two-tiered system. PHC is the first tier and second tier is the urban health organization at the level of the Govt. general hospital, where reference is made from the primary center.
13. **Mental health:** A network of decentralized mental health services for ameliorating categories of disorders starting from PHC, where general duty doctor would be able to prescribed medicine. Upgrading of the physical infrastructure of such institutions at central Govt. expense is also emphasized.
14. **Information, education and communication:** Maximizes IEC to these population group can be achieved not only by mass media, but also by interpersonal communication, folk media involving PRIs/NGOs/Trusts.
15. **Health research:** Increase in Govt funded health research to a level of 1 percent of the total health spending in 2005. Up to 2 percent in 2010 for domestic medical research focusing on new therapeutic drugs and vaccine for tropical diseases, such as TB, malaria, HIV/AIDS.
16. **Role of the private sector:** The policy welcomes participation of the private sector in all areas of health activities. Established legislation for regulating minimum infrastructure and quality standard in clinical establishment of medical institution. Other prescriptions are:
    - National disease surveillance network
    - Health statistics establishment/medical institution
    - Women's health
    - Medical ethics
    - Enforcement of quality standards for food and drugs
    - Regulation of standards in paramedical disciplines
    - Environmental and occupational health
    - Providing medical facilities to users from overseas
    - National Health and Family Welfare Program in India
    - National ARI Program
    - Revised National Tuberculosis Program
    - National Antimalaria Program
    - National Filarial Control Program
    - National Guinea Worm Eradication Program
    - National Leprosy Eradication Program
    - National AIDS Control Program
    - STD Control Program
    - National Program for Control of Blindness
    - Iodine Deficiency Disorder Program
    - Expanded Program on Immunization
    - National Family Welfare Program–RCH Program Historical Development, Organization, Administration, Research, Constraints.
    - National Water Supply and Sanitation Program
    - Minimum Need Program
    - National Diabetes Control Program
    - Polio Eradication Pulse Polio Program
    - National Nutrition Anemia Prophylaxis Program
    - Twenty-point Program

- ICDS Program
- Mid-day Meal Applied Nutritional Program
- National Mental Health Program
- National Health Agency
- Indian Red Cross
- Indian Council for Child Welfare
- Family Planning Association of India
- Tuberculosis Association of India
- Hindkusht Nivaran Sangh
- Central Social Welfare Board
- All India Women Conference
- Blind Association of India.

# NATIONAL HEALTH PROGRAMS

## INTRODUCTION

Since India became independent, the national government has launched a number of health programs to solve the national health problems and improve the health of the people. Most of these programs have been aided by International Agencies such as the WHO, UNICEF and USAID.

## NATIONAL ANTI-MALARIAL PROGRAM

In 1953, National Malaria Control Program began. Because of the spectacular success achieved in the control of malaria, the control program was converted in 1958 into an eradication program with the object of eradicating malaria once and for all from the country. There is a sharp increase in malaria incidence in 1976. In 1977, Govt. of India evolved a modified plan of operation-based effective control rather than eradication.

In 1994, Malaria Action Program was evolved by Govt. of India to appoint an expert committee on malaria to identify the problem areas and to suggest specific measures against malaria.

### Objectives

- Management of serious and complicated malaria cases;
- Prevention of mortality with particular reference to high-risk groups;
- Reduction of morbidity;
- Control of outbreak of epidemics
- Reduction of *Plasmodium falciparum* incidence and containment of drug resistance malaria;
- Maintenance of low-incidence status (Antimalaria month-June)

## NATIONAL FILARIA CONTROL PROGRAM

This was launched in 1955.

### Activities

- Anti-mosquito and antilevel measures in endemic areas
- Establishment of filarial clinics for the detection and treatment of positive microfilaria cases
- Provision of underground drainage in hyper-endemic cities and towns
- Since 1978, the operational component of the NFCP has been merged with the urban malarial scheme, but the research and activities continue to be with Director, National Institute of Communicable Diseases, Delhi.

## NATIONAL TUBERCULOSIS CONTROL PROGRAM

It is a centrally sponsored program.

### Activities

- Early detection and domiciliary treatment of TB cases
- BCG vaccination of infants and children
- Isolation facility especially to those, who require surgery and emergency treatment
- Training and demonstration
- Rehabilitation
- Research
- In 1962, District Tuberculosis Control Program was evolved as a new approach to the community control of tuberculosis.
- In 1993, WHO declared tuberculosis as a global emergency direct observed treatment, short course (DOTS) is recommended strategy for global tuberculosis control.

## NATIONAL LEPORSY ERADICATION PROGRAM

### Objective

Early detection of leprosy cases and their treatment (domiciliary) with multidrug therapy to control the spread of leprosy.

### Units

- National Leprosy Control Units
- Established in highly endemic areas
- Covers population of 4 lakhs
- Headed by a medical officer under whom 20 paramedical workers
- Two non-medical supervisors for 10 PMWs.
- Survey, education and treatment centers.
- Covers a population of 25,000
- Looked after by a PMW who work under the guidance of the medical officer of the primary health center.

## NATIONAL AIDS CONTROL PROGRAM

This program was launched in India in the year 1987. The Ministry of Health and Family Welfare has set up National AIDS Control Organization as separate wing of the program.

### Aims

- To prevent further transmission of HIV
- To decrease morbidity and mortality associated with HIV infection
- To minimize the socioeconomic impact resulting from HIV infection.

### Components

- Establishment of surveillance centers to cover the whole country
- Identification of high-risk groups and their screening
- Issuing specific guidelines for management of detected cases and their follow-up
- Formulating guidelines for blood banks.

# ASSIGNMENT–26 (A): HEALTH EDUCATION

Deliver health education: ____________________

Topic: ____________________

Group: ____________________

Size of group: ____________________

Venue: ____________________

Date: ____________________

Time: ____________________

Previous knowledge: ____________________

Method of teaching: ____________________

AV aids: ____________________

General objectives: ____________________

| Time | Specific objectives | Content | Teaching and learning activities | AV aids | Evaluation |
|---|---|---|---|---|---|
| | | | | | |

| Time | Specific objectives | Content | Teaching and learning activities | AV aids | Evaluation |
|---|---|---|---|---|---|
| | | | | | |

| Time | Specific objectives | Content | Teaching and learning activities | AV aids | Evaluation |
|---|---|---|---|---|---|
| | | | | | |

| Time | Specific objectives | Content | Teaching and learning activities | AV aids | Evaluation |
|---|---|---|---|---|---|
| | | | | | |

| Time | Specific objectives | Content | Teaching and learning activities | AV aids | Evaluation |
|---|---|---|---|---|---|
| | | | | | |

| Time | Specific objectives | Content | Teaching and learning activities | AV aids | Evaluation |
|---|---|---|---|---|---|
| | | | | | |

## EVALUATION FOR HEALTH TALK

Name ____________________

Audience ____________________ Date ____________________

No. of Audience ____________________ Time ____________________

Topic ____________________ Place ____________________

Total marks ____________________

| Sl. No. | Factors/Elements | 1 | 2 | 3 | 4 | 5 |
|---|---|---|---|---|---|---|
| 1. | The Student's personal appearance | So-so | Improbable | Satisfactory | Good | Excellent |
| 2. | Poise | Seldom appeared | Some tension apparent | Yes/No | Most of the time | Always |
| 3. | Voice and clarity | Monotonous | Dull | Satisfactory | Pleasant | Lively |
| 4 | Distractive gestures/ mannerism | Almost/always | Usually | Sometimes | Not very often | Hardly ever |
| **Content and presentation** | | | | | | |
| 5. | Amount of material | Nothing worth-while | Too much | Satisfactory | Well-planned | Very well-planned and presented |
| 6. | Organization and explanation | Could not understand | Difficult to follow | Fairly clear | Clear | Very clear and easy to follow |
| 7. | Environment | Not considered important | Just thought of satisfactory | Organized: satisfactory sometimes | Well-organized | Very well planned |
| 8. | Impressiveness | Practically nil | Occasionlly just clear | appropriate | Good | Very good very appropriate |
| 9. | AV aids Black-board | Too crowded illegible | Untidy partly illegible | Satisfactory | Materials logically appropriate | Very well-maintained appropriate |
| 10. | Diagram, charts, and models | Not planned not prepared | Just appropriate | Satisfactory | Appropriate | Very clear and informative |

**Teacher's sign**

## ASSIGNMENT–26 (B): HEALTH EDUCATION

Deliver a health education the topic: ______________________________

Topic: ______________________________

Group: ______________________________

Size of group: ______________________________

Venue: ______________________________

Date: ______________________________

Time: ______________________________

Previous knowledge: ______________________________

Method of teaching: ______________________________

AV aids: ______________________________

General objectives: ______________________________

| Time | Specific objectives | Content | Teaching and learning activities | AV aids | Evaluation |
|---|---|---|---|---|---|
| | | | | | |

| Time | Specific objectives | Content | Teaching and learning activities | AV aids | Evaluation |
|---|---|---|---|---|---|
| | | | | | |

| Time | Specific objectives | Content | Teaching and learning activities | AV aids | Evaluation |
|---|---|---|---|---|---|
| | | | | | |

| Time | Specific objectives | Content | Teaching and learning activities | AV aids | Evaluation |
|---|---|---|---|---|---|
| | | | | | |

| Time | Specific objectives | Content | Teaching and learning activities | AV aids | Evaluation |
|---|---|---|---|---|---|
| | | | | | |

# EVALUATION FOR HEALTH TALK

Name: ______________________________

Audience: ______________ Date: ______________

No. of Audience: ______________ Time: ______________

Topic: ______________ Place: ______________

Total marks: ______________

| Sl. No. | Factors/Elements | 1 | 2 | 3 | 4 | 5 |
|---|---|---|---|---|---|---|
| 1. | The student's personal appearance | So-so | Improbable | Satisfactory | Good | Excellent |
| 2. | Poise | Seldom appeared | Some tension apparent | Yes/No | Most of the time | Always |
| 3. | Voice and clarity | Monotonous | Dull | Satisfactory | Pleasant | Lively |
| 4 | Distractive gestures/ mannerism | Almost/always | Usually | Sometimes | Not very often | Hardly ever |
| **Content and presentation** | | | | | | |
| 5. | Amount of material | Nothing worthwhile | Too much | Satisfactory | Well-planned | Very well-planned and presented |
| 6. | Organization and explanation | Could not understand | Difficult to follow | Fairly clear | Clear | Very clear and easy to follow |
| 7. | Environment | Not considered important | Just thought of satisfactory | Organized/ satisfactory sometimes | Well-organized | Very well planned |
| 8. | Impressiveness | Practically nil | Occasionally just clear | Appropriate | Good | Very good, very appropriate |
| 9. | AV aids black-board | Too crowded illegible | Untidy partly illegible | Satisfactory | Materials logically appropriate | Very well-maintained appropriate |
| 10. | Diagram, charts, and models | Not planned not prepared | Just appropriate | Satisfactory | Appropriate | Very clear informative |

**Teacher's sign**

## ASSIGNMENT–26 (C): HEALTH EDUCATION

Deliver health education: ________________

Topic: ________________

Group: ________________

Size of group: ________________

Venue: ________________

Date: ________________

Time: ________________

Previous knowledge: ________________

Method of teaching: ________________

AV aids: ________________

General objectives: ________________

| Time | Specific objectives | Content | Teaching and learning activities | AV aids | Evaluation |
|---|---|---|---|---|---|
| | | | | | |

| Time | Specific objectives | Content | Teaching and learning activities | AV aids | Evaluation |
|---|---|---|---|---|---|
| | | | | | |

| Time | Specific objectives | Content | Teaching and learning activities | AV aids | Evaluation |
|---|---|---|---|---|---|
| | | | | | |

| Time | Specific objectives | Content | Teaching and learning activities | AV aids | Evaluation |
|---|---|---|---|---|---|
| | | | | | |

| Time | Specific objectives | Content | Teaching and learning activities | AV aids | Evaluation |
|---|---|---|---|---|---|
| | | | | | |

## EVALUATION FOR HEALTH TALK

Name: ____________________

Audience: ____________ Date: ____________

No. of audience: ____________ Time: ____________

Topic: ____________ Place: ____________

Total marks: ____________

| Sl. No. | Factors/Elements | 1 | 2 | 3 | 4 | 5 |
|---|---|---|---|---|---|---|
| 1. | The student's personal appearance | So-so | Improbable | Satisfactory | Good | Excellent |
| 2. | Poise | Seldom appeared | Some tension apparent | Yes/No | Most of the time | Always |
| 3. | Voice and clarity | Monotonous | Dull | Satisfactory | Pleasant | Lively |
| 4. | Distractive gestures/mannerism | Almost/always | Usually | Sometimes | Not very often | Hardly ever |
| **Content and presentation** | | | | | | |
| 5. | Amount of material | Nothing worthwhile | Too much | Satisfactory | Well- planned | Very well-planned and presented |
| 6. | Organization and explanation | Could not understand | Difficult to follow | Fairly clear | Clear | Very clear and easy to follow |
| 7. | Environment | Not considered as so important | Just thought of satisfactory | Organized satisfactory sometimes | Well organized | Very well planned |
| 8. | Impressiveness | Practically nil | Occasionlly just clear | Appropriate | Good | Very good, very appropriate |
| 9. | AV aids—Blackboard | Too crowded illegible | Untidy partly illegible | Satisfactory | Materials logically appropriate | Very well maintained, appropriate |
| 10. | Diagram, charts and models | Not planned, not prepared | Just appropriate | Satisfactory | Appropriate | Very clear informative |

**Teacher's sign**

## ASSIGNMENT–26 (D): HEALTH EDUCATION

Deliver health education ____________________

Topic: ____________________

Group: ____________________

Size of group: ____________________

Venue: ____________________

Date: ____________________

Time: ____________________

Previous knowledge: ____________________

Method of teaching: ____________________

AV aids: ____________________

General objectives: ____________________

| Time | Specific objectives | Content | Teaching and learning activities | AV aids | Evaluation |
|---|---|---|---|---|---|
| | | | | | |

| Time | Specific objectives | Content | Teaching and learning activities | AV aids | Evaluation |
|---|---|---|---|---|---|
| | | | | | |

| Time | Specific objectives | Content | Teaching and learning activities | AV aids | Evaluation |
|---|---|---|---|---|---|
| | | | | | |

| Time | Specific objectives | Content | Teaching and learning activities | AV aids | Evaluation |
|---|---|---|---|---|---|
| | | | | | |

| Time | Specific objectives | Content | Teaching and learning activities | AV aids | Evaluation |
|---|---|---|---|---|---|
| | | | | | |

## EVALUATION FOR HEALTH TALK

Name: ____________________

Audience: ____________ Date: ____________

No. of audience: ____________ Time: ____________

Topic: ____________ Place: ____________

Total marks: ____________

| Sl. No. | Factors/Elements | 1 | 2 | 3 | 4 | 5 |
|---|---|---|---|---|---|---|
| 1. | The student's personal appearance | So-so | Improbable | Satisfactory | Good | Excellent |
| 2. | Poise | Seldom appeared | Some tension apparent | Yes/No | Most of the time | Always |
| 3. | Voice and clarity | Monotonous | Dull | Satisfactory | Pleasant | Lively |
| 4. | Distractive gestures/mannerism | Almost/always | Usually | Sometimes | Not very often | Hardly ever |
| **Content and presentation** | | | | | | |
| 5. | Amount of material | Nothing worthwhile | Too much | Satisfactory | Well-planned | Very well-planned and presented |
| 6. | Organization and explanation | Could not understand | Difficult to follow | Fairly clear | Clear | Very clear and easy to follow |
| 7. | Environment | Not considered important | Just thought of satisfactory | Organized satisfactory sometimes | Well-organized | Very well planned |
| 8. | Impressiveness | Practically nil | Occasionlly just clear | appropriate | Good | Very good, very appropriate |
| 9. | AV aids Blackboard | Too crowded illegible | Untidy partly illegible | Satisfactory | Materials logically appropriate | Very well-maintained, appropriate |
| 10. | Diagram, charts and models | Not planned, not prepared | Just appropriate | Satisfactory | Appropriate | Very clear and informative |

**Teacher's sign**

## ASSIGNMENT–26 (E): HEALTH EDUCATION

Deliver health education ______________________________

Topic: ______________________________

Group: ______________________________

Size of group: ______________________________

Venue: ______________________________

Date: ______________________________

Time: ______________________________

Previous knowledge: ______________________________

Method of teaching: ______________________________

AV aids: ______________________________

General objectives: ______________________________

| Time | Specific objectives | Content | Teaching and learning activities | AV aids | Evaluation |
|---|---|---|---|---|---|
| | | | | | |

| Time | Specific objectives | Content | Teaching and learning activities | AV aids | Evaluation |
|---|---|---|---|---|---|
| | | | | | |

| Time | Specific objectives | Content | Teaching and learning activities | AV aids | Evaluation |
|---|---|---|---|---|---|
| | | | | | |

| Time | Specific objectives | Content | Teaching and learning activities | AV aids | Evaluation |
|---|---|---|---|---|---|
| | | | | | |

| Time | Specific objectives | Content | Teaching and learning activities | AV aids | Evaluation |
|---|---|---|---|---|---|
| | | | | | |

## EVALUATION FOR HEALTH TALK

Name: ______________________________

Audience: ______________ Date: ______________

No. of audience: ______________ Time: ______________

Topic: ______________ Place: ______________

Total marks: ______________

| Sl. No. | Factors/Elements | 1 | 2 | 3 | 4 | 5 |
|---|---|---|---|---|---|---|
| 1. | The student's personal appearance | So-so | Improbable | Satisfactory | Good | Excellent |
| 2. | Poise | Seldom appeared | Some tension apparent | Yes/No | Most of the time | Always |
| 3. | Voice and clarity | Monotonous | Dull | Satisfactory | Pleasant | Lively |
| 4. | Distractive gestures/ mannerism | Almost/always | Usually | Sometimes | Not very often | Hardly ever |
| **Content and Presentation** | | | | | | |
| 5. | Amount of material | Nothing worthwhile | Too much | Satisfactory | Well-planned | Very well-planned and presented |
| 6. | Organization and explanation | Could not understand | Difficult to follow | Fairly clear | Clear | Very clear and easy to follow |
| 7. | Environment | Not considered as so important | Just thought of satisfactory | Organized satisfactory sometimes | Well-organized | Very well planned |
| 8. | Impressiveness | Practically nil | Occasionlly just clear | Appropriate | Good | Very good, very appropriate |
| 9. | AV aids Blackboard | Too crowded illegible | Untidy partly illegible | Satisfactory | Materials logically appropriate | Very well-maintained, appropriate |
| 10. | Diagram, charts and models | Not planned not prepared | Just appropriate | Satisfactory | Appropriate | Very clear and informative |

**Teacher's sign**

# 9. FIELD VISIT

## ASSIGNMENT–27 (A): OBSERVATION REPORT

### Field Visit to a Community Health Agency

**Field visit report for the:**

- Old age home
- Orphanage
- Home for physically, mentally and socially challenged, home for destitute
- Child guidance clinic
- Trauma units
- Well-baby clinic, etc.

Write an observation report of a community health agency you visited, using the following guidelines.

Name of the agency: ______________________________
Date of visit: ______________________________

1. Where is this institute located? ____________________

2. When, where and how did this institute originate?

3. List down the objectives of this institute.

4. What are the functions of institute?

5. Mention the various departments existing in the institute.

6. Draw its organizational structure.

7. Draw the organizational pattern of nursing departments.

8. What is the staffing pattern and duty timings for the nurses at the institution?

9. Briefly describe about the physical setup of institution.

10. Give a brief account of learning experience achieved from this visit.

# ASSIGNMENT–27 (B): OBSERVATION REPORT

## Field Visit to a Community Health Agency

**Field visit report for the:**

- Old age home
- Orphanage
- Home for physically, mentally and socially challenged, home for destitute
- Child guidance clinic
- Trauma units
- Well-baby clinic, etc.

Write an observation report of a community health agency you visited, using the following guidelines.

Name of the agency: ________________________

Date of visit: ________________________

1. Where is this institute located? ________________________

2. When, where and how did this institute originate?

3. List down the objectives of this institute.

4. What are the functions of this institute?

5. Mention the various departments existing in the institute.

6. Draw its organizational structure.

7. Draw the organizational pattern of nursing departments.

8. What is the staffing pattern and duty timings for the nurses at the institution?

9. Briefly describe about the physical setup of institution.

10. Give a brief account of learning experience achieved from this visit.

# ASSIGNMENT–27 (C): OBSERVATION REPORTS

## Field Visit to a Community Health Agency

**Field visit report for the:**

- Old age homes
- Orphanage
- Home for physically, mentally and socially challenged, home for destitute
- Child guidance clinic
- Trauma units
- Well-baby clinic, etc.

Write an observation report of a community health agency you visited, using the following guidelines.

Name of the agency: ______________________

Date of visit: ______________________

1. Where is this institute located? ______________________

2. When, where and how did this institute originate?

3. List down the objectives of this institute.

4. What are the functions of the institute?

5. Mention the various departments existing in the institute.

6. Draw its organizational structure.

7. Draw the organizational pattern of nursing departments.

8. What is the staffing pattern and duty timings for the nurses at the institution?

9. Briefly describe about the physical setup of institution.

10. Give a brief account of learning experience achieved from this visit.

# ASSIGNMENT–27 (D): OBSERVATION REPORTS

## Field Visit to a Community Health Agency

**Field visit report for the:**

- Old age home
- Orphanage
- Home for physically, mentally and socially challenged home for destitute
- Child guidance clinic
- Trauma units,
- Well-baby clinic, etc.

Write an observation report of a community health agency you visited, using the following guidelines.

Name of the agency: ______________________________

Date of visit: ______________________________

1. Where is this institute located? ______________________________

2. When, where and how did this institute originate?

3. List down the objectives of this institute.

4. What are the functions of the institute?

5. Mention the various departments existing in the institute.

6. Draw its organizational structure.

7. Draw the organizational pattern of nursing departments.

8. What is the staffing pattern and duty timings for the nurses at the institution?

9. Briefly describe about the physical setup of institution.

10. Give a brief account of learning experience achieved from this visit.

## ASSIGNMENT–27 (E): OBSERVATION REPORT

### Field Visit to a Community Health Agency

**Field visit report for the:**

- Old age home
- Orphanage
- Home for physically, mentally and socially challenged, home for destitute
- Child guidance clinic
- Trauma units
- Well-baby clinic, etc.

Write an observation report of a community health agency you visited, using the following guidelines.

Name of the agency: ____________________

Date of visit: ____________________

1. Where is this institute located? ____________________

2. When, where and how did this institute originate?

3. List down the objectives of this institute.

4. What are the functions of the institute?

5. Mention the various departments existing in the institute.

6. Draw its organizational structure.

7. Draw the organizational pattern of nursing departments.

8. What is the staffing pattern and duty timings for the nurses at the institution?

9. Briefly describe about the physical setup of institution.

10. Give a brief account of learning experience achieved from this visit.

# 10. BAG TECHNIQUE

## Definition

Bag technique is a tool making use of public health bag through which the nurse, during his/her home visit, can perform nursing procedures with ease and deftness, saving time and effort with the end in view of rendering effective nursing care.

Public health bag is an essential and indispensable equipment of the public health nurse, which he/she has to carry along when he/she goes out on home visiting. It contains basic medications and articles, which are necessary for giving care.

## Rationale

To render effective nursing care to clients and/or members of the family during home visit.

## Principles

The use of the bag technique should minimize, if not totally prevents, the spread of infection from individuals to families, hence, to the community.

Bag technique should save time and effort on the part of the nurse in the performance of nursing procedures. It should not overshadow concern for the patient rather should show the effectiveness of total care given to an individual or family. It can be performed in a variety of ways depending upon agency policies, actual home situation, etc. as long as principles of avoiding transfer of infection is carried out.

## Special Considerations in the Use of the Bag

The bag should contain all necessary articles, supplies and equipment, which may be used to answer emergency needs. The bag and its contents should be cleaned as often as possible, supplies replaced and ready for use at any time.

The bag and its contents should be well protected from contact with any article in the home of the patients. Consider the bag and its contents clean and/or sterile, while any article belonging to the patient as dirty and contaminated.

The arrangement of the contents of the bag should be the one most convenient to the user to facilitate the efficiency and avoid confusion.

Handwashing is done as frequently as the situation calls for, helps in minimizing or avoiding contamination of the bag and its contents.

The bag when used for a communicable case should be thoroughly cleaned and disinfected before keeping and reusing.

## Contents of the Bag

- Paper lining
- Extra paper for making bag for waste materials (paper bag)
- Plastic linen/lining
- Apron
- Hand towel in plastic bag

- Soap in soap dish
- Thermometers in case (1 oral and rectal)
- Two pairs of scissors (1 surgical and 1 bandage)
- Two pairs of forceps (curved and straight)
- Syringes (5 mL and 2 mL)
- Hypodermic needles g. 19, 22, 23, 25
- Sterile dressings (OS, CB)
- Sterile cord tie
- Adhesive plaster
- Dressing (OS, cotton ball)
- Alcohol lamp
- Tape measure
- Baby's scale
- One pair of rubber gloves
- Two test tubes
- Test tube holder
- Medicines
- Betadine
- 70% alcohol
- Ophthalmic ointment (antibiotic)
- Zephiran solution
- Hydrogen peroxide
- Spirit of ammonia
- Acetic acid
- Benedict's solution

**Note:** Blood pressure apparatus and stethoscope are carried separately.

## Steps/Procedures

Actions Rationale

1. Upon arriving at the client's home, place the bag on the table or any flat surface lined with paper lining, clean side out (folded part touching the table). Put the bag's handles or strap beneath the bag.
   To protect the bag from contamination.
2. Ask for a basin of water and a glass of water if faucet is not available. Place these outside the work area. To be used for handwashing.
   To protect the work field from being wet.
3. Open the bag, take the linen/plastic lining and spread over work field or area. The paper lining, clean side out (folded part out). To make a non-contaminated work field or area.
4. Take out hand towel, soap dish and apron and the place them at one corner of the work area (within the confines of the linen/plastic lining). To prepare for handwashing.
5. Do handwashing. Wipe, dry with towel. Leave the plastic wrappers of the towel in a soap dish in the bag. Handwashing prevents possible infection from one care provider to the client.
5. Put on apron right side out and wrong side with crease touching the body, sliding the head into the neck strap. Neatly tie the straps at the back. To protect the nurses' uniform.
6. Put out things most needed for the specific case, e.g., thermometer, kidney basin, cotton ball, waste paper bag) and place at one corner of the work area. To make them readily accessible.
7. Place waste paper bag outside of work area. To prevent contamination of clean area.
8. Close the bag. To give comfort and security, maintain personal hygiene and hasten recovery.
9. Proceed to the specific nursing care or treatment. To prevent contamination of bag and contents.
10. After completing nursing care or treatment, clean and alcoholize the things used. To protect caregiver and prevent spread of infection to others.
11. Do handwashing again.

12. Open the bag and put back all articles in their proper places.
13. Remove apron folding away from the body, with soiled sidefolded inwards, and the clean side out. Place it in the bag.
14. Fold the linen/plastic lining, clean; place it in the bag and close the bag.
15. Make post-visit conference on matters relevant to health care, taking anecdotal notes preparatory to final reporting. To be used as reference for future visit.
16. Make appointment for the next visit (either home or clinic), taking note of the date, time and purpose for follow-up care.

## After Care

1. Before keeping all articles in the bag, clean and alcoholize them.
2. Get the bag from the table, fold the paper lining (and insert) and place in between the flaps and cover the bag. Evaluation and Documentation
3. Record all relevant findings about the client and members of the family.
4. Take note of environmental factors, which affect the clients/family health.
5. Include quality of nurse-patient relationship.
6. Assess effectiveness of nursing care provided.

## ASSIGNMENT–28 (A): BAG TECHNIQUE PROCEDURE

(BAG TECHNIQUE)

### LESSON PLAN

Name of student teacher: ____________________

Subject: ____________________

Topic: ____________________

Group: ____________________

Date: ____________________

Time: ____________________

Place: ____________________

Method of teaching: ____________________

Teaching aids: ____________________

Previous knowledge: ____________________

### OBJECTIVES

General Objectives

Specific Objectives

| Sl. No. | Specific objectives | Content matter | Method of teaching | AV aids | Teaching and learning activity | Evaluation |
|---|---|---|---|---|---|---|
| | | | | | | |

| Sl. No. | Specific objectives | Content matter | Method of teaching | AV aids | Teaching and learning activity | Evaluation |
|---|---|---|---|---|---|---|
| | | | | | | |

| Sl. No. | Specific objectives | Content matter | Method of teaching | AV aids | Teaching and learning activity | Evaluation |
|---|---|---|---|---|---|---|
| | | | | | | |

| Sl. No. | Specific objectives | Content matter | Method of teaching | AV aids | Teaching and learning activity | Evaluation |
|---|---|---|---|---|---|---|
| | | | | | | |

**Bibliography**

# ASSIGNMENT–28 (B): BAG TECHNIQUE PROCEDURE

(HOME VISIT)

## LESSON PLAN

Name of student teacher: ______

Subject: ______

Topic: ______

Group: ______

Date: ______

Time: ______

Place: ______

Method of teaching: ______

Teaching aids: ______

Previous knowledge: ______

## OBJECTIVES

General Objectives

______

Specific Objectives

______

| Sl. No. | Specific objectives | Content matter | Method of teaching | AV aids | Teaching and learning activity | Evaluation |
|---|---|---|---|---|---|---|
| | | | | | | |

| Sl. No. | Specific objectives | Content matter | Method of teaching | AV aids | Teaching and learning activity | Evaluation |
|---|---|---|---|---|---|---|
| | | | | | | |

| Sl. No. | Specific objectives | Content matter | Method of teaching | AV aids | Teaching and learning activity | Evaluation |
|---|---|---|---|---|---|---|
| | | | | | | |

| Sl. No. | Specific objectives | Content matter | Method of teaching | AV aids | Teaching and learning activity | Evaluation |
|---|---|---|---|---|---|---|
| | | | | | | |

**Bibliography**

## ASSIGNMENT–28 (C): BAG TECHNIQUE PROCEDURE

(HANDWASHING)

### LESSON PLAN

Name of student teacher: ____________________

Subject: ____________________

Topic: ____________________

Group: ____________________

Date: ____________________

Time: ____________________

Place ____________________

Method of teaching: ____________________

Teaching aids: ____________________

Previous knowledge: ____________________

### OBJECTIVES

General Objectives

Specific Objectives

| Sl. No. | Specific objectives | Content matter | Method of teaching | AV aids | Teaching and learning activity | Evaluation |
|---|---|---|---|---|---|---|
| | | | | | | |

| Sl. No. | Specific objectives | Content matter | Method of teaching | AV aids | Teaching and learning activity | Evaluation |
|---|---|---|---|---|---|---|
| | | | | | | |

| Sl. No. | Specific objectives | Content matter | Method of teaching | AV aids | Teaching and learning activity | Evaluation |
|---|---|---|---|---|---|---|
| | | | | | | |

| Sl. No. | Specific objectives | Content matter | Method of teaching | AV aids | Teaching and learning activity | Evaluation |
|---|---|---|---|---|---|---|
| | | | | | | |

**Bibliography**

# ASSIGNMENT–28 (D): BAG TECHNIQUE PROCEDURE

(TEMPERATURE TECHNIQUE)

## LESSON PLAN

Name of student teacher: ____________________

Subject: ____________________

Topic: ____________________

Group: ____________________

Date: ____________________

Time: ____________________

Place ____________________

Method of teaching: ____________________

Teaching aids: ____________________

Previous knowledge: ____________________

## OBJECTIVES

General Objectives

Specific Objectives

| Sl. No. | Specific objectives | Content matter | Method of teaching | AV aids | Teaching and learning activity | Evaluation |
|---|---|---|---|---|---|---|
| | | | | | | |

| Sl. No. | Specific objectives | Content matter | Method of teaching | AV aids | Teaching and learning activity | Evaluation |
|---|---|---|---|---|---|---|
| | | | | | | |

| Sl. No. | Specific objectives | Content matter | Method of teaching | AV aids | Teaching and learning activity | Evaluation |
|---|---|---|---|---|---|---|
| | | | | | | |

| Sl. No. | Specific objectives | Content matter | Method of teaching | AV aids | Teaching and learning activity | Evaluation |
|---|---|---|---|---|---|---|
| | | | | | | |

**Bibliography**

# ASSIGNMENT–28 (E): BAG TECHNIQUE PROCEDURE

(WOUND DRESSING)

## LESSON PLAN

Name of student teacher: ____________________

Subject: ____________________

Topic: ____________________

Group: ____________________

Date: ____________________

Time: ____________________

Place: ____________________

Method of teaching: ____________________

Teaching aids: ____________________

Previous knowledge: ____________________

## OBJECTIVES

General Objectives

Specific Objectives

| Sl. No. | Specific objectives | Content matter | Method of teaching | AV aids | Teaching and learning activity | Evaluation |
|---|---|---|---|---|---|---|
| | | | | | | |

| Sl. No. | Specific objectives | Content matter | Method of teaching | AV aids | Teaching and learning activity | Evaluation |
|---|---|---|---|---|---|---|
| | | | | | | |

| Sl. No. | Specific objectives | Content matter | Method of teaching | AV aids | Teaching and learning activity | Evaluation |
|---|---|---|---|---|---|---|
| | | | | | | |

| Sl. No. | Specific objectives | Content matter | Method of teaching | AV aids | Teaching and learning activity | Evaluation |
| --- | --- | --- | --- | --- | --- | --- |
| | | | | | | |

**Bibliography**

# ASSIGNMENT–28 (F): BAG TECHNIQUE PROCEDURE

(ANTENATAL CARE)

## LESSON PLAN

Name of student teacher: ____________________

Subject: ____________________

Topic: ____________________

Group: ____________________

Date: ____________________

Time: ____________________

Place: ____________________

Method of teaching: ____________________

Teaching aids: ____________________

Previous knowledge: ____________________

## OBJECTIVES

General Objectives

____________________

____________________

____________________

Specific Objectives

____________________

____________________

____________________

____________________

____________________

____________________

____________________

____________________

____________________

____________________

____________________

____________________

____________________

____________________

____________________

____________________

____________________

____________________

____________________

| Sl. No. | Specific objectives | Content matter | Method of teaching | AV aids | Teaching and learning activity | Evaluation |
|---|---|---|---|---|---|---|
| | | | | | | |

| Sl. No. | Specific objectives | Content matter | Method of teaching | AV aids | Teaching and learning activity | Evaluation |
|---|---|---|---|---|---|---|
| | | | | | | |

| Sl. No. | Specific objectives | Content matter | Method of teaching | AV aids | Teaching and learning activity | Evaluation |
|---|---|---|---|---|---|---|
| | | | | | | |

| Sl. No. | Specific objectives | Content matter | Method of teaching | AV aids | Teaching and learning activity | Evaluation |
|---|---|---|---|---|---|---|
| | | | | | | |

**Bibliography**

## ASSIGNMENT–28 (G): BAG TECHNIQUE PROCEDURE

(URINE TESTING)

### LESSON PLAN

Name of student teacher: ____________________

Subject: ____________________

Topic: ____________________

Group: ____________________

Date: ____________________

Time: ____________________

Place: ____________________

Method of teaching: ____________________

Teaching aids: ____________________

Previous knowledge: ____________________

### OBJECTIVES

General Objectives

Specific Objectives

| Sl. No. | Specific objectives | Content matter | Method of teaching | AV aids | Teaching and learning activity | Evaluation |
|---|---|---|---|---|---|---|
| | | | | | | |

| Sl. No. | Specific objectives | Content matter | Method of teaching | AV aids | Teaching and learning activity | Evaluation |
|---|---|---|---|---|---|---|
| | | | | | | |

| Sl. No. | Specific objectives | Content matter | Method of teaching | AV aids | Teaching and learning activity | Evaluation |
|---|---|---|---|---|---|---|
| | | | | | | |

| Sl. No. | Specific objectives | Content matter | Method of teaching | AV aids | Teaching and learning activity | Evaluation |
|---|---|---|---|---|---|---|
| | | | | | | |

**Bibliography**

# ASSIGNMENT–28 (H): BAG TECHNIQUE PROCEDURE

(POSTNATAL CARE)

## LESSON PLAN

Name of student teacher: ____________________

Subject: ____________________

Topic: ____________________

Group: ____________________

Date: ____________________

Time: ____________________

Place: ____________________

Method of teaching: ____________________

Teaching aids: ____________________

Previous knowledge: ____________________

## OBJECTIVES

General Objectives

Specific Objectives

| Sl. No. | Specific objectives | Content matter | Method of teaching | AV aids | Teaching and learning activity | Evaluation |
|---|---|---|---|---|---|---|
| | | | | | | |

| Sl. No. | Specific objectives | Content matter | Method of teaching | AV aids | Teaching and learning activity | Evaluation |
|---|---|---|---|---|---|---|
| | | | | | | |

| Sl. No. | Specific objectives | Content matter | Method of teaching | AV aids | Teaching and learning activity | Evaluation |
|---|---|---|---|---|---|---|
| | | | | | | |

| Sl. No. | Specific objectives | Content matter | Method of teaching | AV aids | Teaching and learning activity | Evaluation |
|---|---|---|---|---|---|---|
| | | | | | | |

**Bibliography**

## ASSIGNMENT–28 (I): BAG TECHNIQUE PROCEDURE

(CORD CARE)

### LESSON PLAN

Name of student teacher: ____________________

Subject: ____________________

Topic: ____________________

Group: ____________________

Date: ____________________

Time: ____________________

Place ____________________

Method of teaching: ____________________

Teaching aids: ____________________

Previous knowledge: ____________________

### OBJECTIVES

General Objectives

Specific Objectives

| Sl. No. | Specific objectives | Content matter | Method of teaching | AV aids | Teaching and learning activity | Evaluation |
|---|---|---|---|---|---|---|
| | | | | | | |

| Sl. No. | Specific objectives | Content matter | Method of teaching | AV aids | Teaching and learning activity | Evaluation |
|---|---|---|---|---|---|---|
| | | | | | | |

| Sl. No. | Specific objectives | Content matter | Method of teaching | AV aids | Teaching and learning activity | Evaluation |
|---|---|---|---|---|---|---|
| | | | | | | |

| Sl. No. | Specific objectives | Content matter | Method of teaching | AV aids | Teaching and learning activity | Evaluation |
|---|---|---|---|---|---|---|
| | | | | | | |

**Bibliography**

# ASSIGNMENT–28 (J): BAG TECHNIQUE PROCEDURE

(EYE IRRIGATION)

## LESSON PLAN

Name of student teacher: ___

Subject: ___

Topic: ___

Group: ___

Date: ___

Time: ___

Place: ___

Method of teaching: ___

Teaching aids: ___

Previous knowledge: ___

## OBJECTIVES

General Objectives

___

Specific Objectives

___

| Sl. No. | Specific objectives | Content matter | Method of teaching | AV aids | Teaching and learning activity | Evaluation |
|---|---|---|---|---|---|---|
| | | | | | | |

| Sl. No. | Specific objectives | Content matter | Method of teaching | AV aids | Teaching and learning activity | Evaluation |
|---|---|---|---|---|---|---|
| | | | | | | |

| Sl. No. | Specific objectives | Content matter | Method of teaching | AV aids | Teaching and learning activity | Evaluation |
|---|---|---|---|---|---|---|
| | | | | | | |

| Sl. No. | Specific objectives | Content matter | Method of teaching | AV aids | Teaching and learning activity | Evaluation |
| --- | --- | --- | --- | --- | --- | --- |
| | | | | | | |

**Bibliography**

# ASSIGNMENT–28 (K): BAG TECHNIQUE PROCEDURE

(BABY BATH)

## LESSON PLAN

Name of student teacher: ____________________

Subject: ____________________

Topic: ____________________

Group: ____________________

Date: ____________________

Time: ____________________

Place: ____________________

Method of teaching: ____________________

Teaching aids: ____________________

Previous knowledge: ____________________

## OBJECTIVES

General Objectives

Specific Objectives

| Sl. No. | Specific objectives | Content matter | Method of teaching | AV aids | Teaching and learning activity | Evaluation |
|---|---|---|---|---|---|---|
| | | | | | | |

| Sl. No. | Specific objectives | Content matter | Method of teaching | AV aids | Teaching and learning activity | Evaluation |
|---|---|---|---|---|---|---|
| | | | | | | |

| Sl. No. | Specific objectives | Content matter | Method of teaching | AV aids | Teaching and learning activity | Evaluation |
|---|---|---|---|---|---|---|
| | | | | | | |

| Sl. No. | Specific objectives | Content matter | Method of teaching | AV aids | Teaching and learning activity | Evaluation |
|---|---|---|---|---|---|---|
| | | | | | | |

**Bibliography**

# ASSIGNMENT–28 (L): BAG TECHNIQUE PROCEDURE

## (UNDER-FIVE ASSESSMENT)

## LESSON PLAN

Name of student teacher: __________

Subject: __________

Topic: __________

Group: __________

Date: __________

Time: __________

Place: __________

Method of teaching: __________

Teaching aids: __________

Previous knowledge: __________

## OBJECTIVES

General Objectives

Specific Objectives

| Sl. No. | Specific objectives | Content matter | Method of teaching | AV aids | Teaching and learning activity | Evaluation |
|---|---|---|---|---|---|---|
| | | | | | | |

| Sl. No. | Specific objectives | Content matter | Method of teaching | AV aids | Teaching and learning activity | Evaluation |
|---|---|---|---|---|---|---|
| | | | | | | |

| Sl. No. | Specific objectives | Content matter | Method of teaching | AV aids | Teaching and learning activity | Evaluation |
|---|---|---|---|---|---|---|
| | | | | | | |

| Sl. No. | Specific objectives | Content matter | Method of teaching | AV aids | Teaching and learning activity | Evaluation |
|---|---|---|---|---|---|---|
| | | | | | | |

**Bibliography**

# ASSIGNMENT–28 (M): BAG TECHNIQUE PROCEDURE

(ORAL REHYDRATION THERAPY)

## LESSON PLAN

Name of student teacher: __________

Subject: __________

Topic: __________

Group: __________

Date: __________

Time: __________

Place: __________

Method of teaching: __________

Teaching aids: __________

Previous knowledge: __________

## OBJECTIVES

General Objectives

Specific Objectives

| Sl. No. | Specific objectives | Content matter | Method of teaching | AV aids | Teaching and learning activity | Evaluation |
|---|---|---|---|---|---|---|
| | | | | | | |

| Sl. No. | Specific objectives | Content matter | Method of teaching | AV aids | Teaching and learning activity | Evaluation |
|---|---|---|---|---|---|---|
| | | | | | | |

| Sl. No. | Specific objectives | Content matter | Method of teaching | AV aids | Teaching and learning activity | Evaluation |
|---|---|---|---|---|---|---|
| | | | | | | |

## Bibliography

# 11. COMMUNITY NURSING PROCESS

## ASSIGNMENT–29 (A): RURAL COMMUNITY

Name: ________________ FF No: ________________

Age: ________________ Date of birth: ________________

1st year/2nd year/3rd year/4th year or ________________ years.

Sex: ________________ Date of care started: ________________

Head of the family: ________________ Date of care ended: ________________

Address: ________________

| Assessment | Goal | Planning | Intervention | Evaluation |
|---|---|---|---|---|
| | | | | |

| Assessment | Goal | Planning | Intervention | Evaluation |
|---|---|---|---|---|
| | | | | |

| Assessment | Goal | Planning | Intervention | Evaluation |
|---|---|---|---|---|
| | | | | |

| Assessment | Goal | Planning | Intervention | Evaluation |
|---|---|---|---|---|
| | | | | |

# ASSIGNMENT–29 (B): RURAL COMMUNITY

Name: ____________________ FF No: ____________________

Age: ____________________ Date of birth: ____________________

1st year/2nd year/3rd year/4th year or ____________________ years.

Sex: ____________________ Date of care started: ____________________

Head of the family: ____________________ Date of care ended: ____________________

Address: ____________________

| Assessment | Goal | Planning | Intervention | Evaluation |
|---|---|---|---|---|
| | | | | |

| Assessment | Goal | Planning | Intervention | Evaluation |
|---|---|---|---|---|
| | | | | |

| Assessment | Goal | Planning | Intervention | Evaluation |
|---|---|---|---|---|
| | | | | |

| Assessment | Goal | Planning | Intervention | Evaluation |
|---|---|---|---|---|
| | | | | |

## ASSIGNMENT–29 (C): URBAN COMMUNITY

Name: ______________________ FF No: ______________________

Age: ______________________ Date of birth: ______________________

1st year/2nd year/3rd year/4th year or ______________________ years.

Sex: ______________________ Date of care started: ______________________

Head of the family: ______________________ Date of care ended: ______________________

Address: ____________________________________________

____________________________________________

____________________________________________

____________________________________________

| Assessment | Goal | Planning | Intervention | Evaluation |
|---|---|---|---|---|
| | | | | |

| Assessment | Goal | Planning | Intervention | Evaluation |
|---|---|---|---|---|
| | | | | |

| Assessment | Goal | Planning | Intervention | Evaluation |
|---|---|---|---|---|
| | | | | |

| Assessment | Goal | Planning | Intervention | Evaluation |
|---|---|---|---|---|
| | | | | |

## ASSIGNMENT–29 (D): URBAN COMMUNITY

Name: ____________________ FF No: ____________________

Age: ____________________ Date of birth: ____________________

1st year/2nd year/3rd year/4th year or ____________________ years.

Sex: ____________________ Date of care started: ____________________

Head of the family: ____________________ Date of care ended: ____________________

Address: ____________________

| Assessment | Goal | Planning | Intervention | Evaluation |
|---|---|---|---|---|
| | | | | |

| Assessment | Goal | Planning | Intervention | Evaluation |
|---|---|---|---|---|
| | | | | |

| Assessment | Goal | Planning | Intervention | Evaluation |
|---|---|---|---|---|
| | | | | |

| Assessment | Goal | Planning | Intervention | Evaluation |
|---|---|---|---|---|
| | | | | |

# 12. SCHOOL HEALTH SERVICES

## INTRODUCTION

School health service is an important branch of community health. According to modern concepts, school health service is an economical and powerful means of raising community health and more important in future generations. The school health service is a personal health service. It has developed during the past 70 years from the narrower concept of medical examination of children to the present-day broader concept of comprehensive care of the health and well-being of children throughout the school years.

## OBJECTIVES

- The promotion of positive health
- The prevention of diseases
- Early diagnosis, treatment and follow-up of defects
- Awakening health consciousness in children
- The provision of healthful environment.

## HEALTH PROBLEMS OF THE SCHOOL CHILD

Any discussion of a school health service must be based on the local health problems of the school child, the culture of the community and the available resources in terms of money, material and manpower. While the health problems of school children vary from one place to another, surveys carried out in India indicate that the main emphasis will fall in the following categories:

- Malnutrition
- Infectious diseases
- Intestinal parasites
- Diseases of skin, eye and ear
- Dental carries.

## ASPECTS OF SCHOOL HEALTH SERVICES

The tasks of a school health service are manifold and vary according to local priorities. Where resources are plentiful, special school health services may be developed. Some aspects of a school health services:

- Health appraisal of school children and school personnel
- Remedial measures and follow-up

- Prevention of communicable diseases
- Healthful school environment
- Nutritional services
- First aid and emergency care
- Mental health
- Dental health
- Eye health
- Health education
- Education of handicapped children
- Proper maintenance and use of school health records.

# ASSIGNMENT–30 (A)

Name of school: ______________________________

Name of pupil: ______________________________

Standard: ______________________________

Age: Years: Sex: M/F

Weight: __________ kg, Height: __________ cm Chest: __________ cm Expansion: __________ cm

General health and nutritional state: ______________________________

Protective inoculations: TAB/vaccination

Physical defects/deformities: ______________________________

CVS ______________________________

Respiratory system: ______________________________

GI system Teeth: ______________________________

Gums: ______________________________

Liver: ______________________________

Spleen: ______________________________

CNS ______________________________

Eyes/vision RE: ______________________________ LE: ______________________________

Ears/hearing RE: ______________________________ LE: ______________________________

Special points

______________________________

______________________________

______________________________

______________________________

______________________________

**School class teaching program**

Deliver a class to school: ______________________________

Topic: ______________________________

Group: ______________________________

Size of group: ______________________________

Date: ______________________________ Time: ______________________________

Previous knowledge: ______________________________

Method of teaching: ______________________________

AV aids: ______________________________

**General objectives:**

**Discuss about the topic:**

**Importance of–**

a. Personal hygiene

b. Environmental hygiene

c. Nutrition

d. Exercise

e. School report
   - Introduction

- Geographical area

- Education level

- Staffs of primary school

- Functions of primary school

- Report of primary school

**Signature of Medical Officer/Principal**

## ASSIGNMENT–30 (B)

Name of school: ___

Name of pupil: ___

Standard: ___

Age: Years: Sex: M/F

Weight: ___ kg, Height: ___ cm Chest: ___ cm Expansion: ___ cm

General health and nutritional state: ___

Protective inoculations: TAB/vaccination

Physical defects/deformities: ___

CVS ___

Respiratory system: ___

GI system Teeth: ___

Gums: ___

Liver: ___

Spleen: ___

CNS ___

Eyes/vision RE: ___ LE: ___

Ears/hearing RE: ___ LE: ___

Special points

___

___

___

___

___

___

**School class teaching program**

Deliver a class to school: ___

Topic: ___

Group: ___

Size of group: ___

Date: ___ Time: ___

Previous knowledge: ___

Method of teaching: ___

AV aids: ___

**General objectives:**

**Discuss about the topic:**

**Importance of –**

a. Personal hygiene

b. Environmental hygiene

c. Nutrition

d. Exercise

e. School report
   - Introduction
   - Geographical area

- Education level

- Staffs of primary school

- Functions of primary school

- Report of primary school

**Signature of Medical Officer/Principal**

# ASSIGNMENT–30 (C)

Name of school: ____________________

Name of pupil: ____________________

Standard: ____________________

Age: Years: Sex: M/F

Weight: __________ kg, Height: __________ cm Chest: __________ cm Expansion: __________ cm

General health and nutritional state: ____________________

Protective inoculations: TAB/vaccination

Physical defects/deformities: ____________________

CVS ____________________

Respiratory system: ____________________

GI system Teeth: ____________________

Gums: ____________________

Liver: ____________________

Spleen: ____________________

CNS ____________________

Eyes/vision RE: ____________________ LE: ____________________

Ears/hearing RE: ____________________ LE: ____________________

Special points

____________________

____________________

____________________

____________________

____________________

____________________

**School class teaching program**

Deliver a class to school: ____________________

Topic: ____________________

Group: ____________________

Size of group: ____________________

Date: ____________________ Time: ____________________

Previous knowledge: ____________________

Method of teaching: ____________________

**General objectives:**

**Discuss about the topic:**

**Importance of—**

a. Personal hygiene

b. Environmental hygiene

c. Nutrition

d. Exercise

e. School report
   - Introduction
   - Geographical area

- Education level

- Staffs of primary school

- Functions of primary school

- Report of primary school

**Signature of Medical Officer/Principal**

# ASSIGNMENT–30 (D)

Name of school: ___

Name of pupil: ___

Standard: ___

Age: Years: Sex: M/F

Weight: ___ kg, Height: ___ cm Chest: ___ cm Expansion: ___ cm

General health and nutritional state: ___

Protective inoculations: TAB/vaccination

Physical defects/deformities: ___

CVS ___

Respiratory system: ___

GI system Teeth: ___

Gums: ___

Liver: ___

Spleen: ___

CNS ___

Eyes/vision RE: ___ LE: ___

Ears/hearing RE: ___ LE: ___

Special points

___

___

___

___

___

___

**School class teaching program**

Deliver a class to school: ___

Topic: ___

Group: ___

Size of group: ___

Date: ___ Time: ___

Previous knowledge: ___

Method of teaching: ___

**General objectives:**

**Discuss about the topic:**

**Importance of —**

a. Personal hygiene

b. Environmental hygiene

c. Nutrition

d. Exercise

e. School report
- Introduction
- Geographical area

- Education level

- Staffs of primary school

- Functions of primary school

- Report of primary school

**Signature of Medical Officer/Principal**

## ASSIGNMENT–30 (E)

Name of school: ____________________

Name of pupil: ____________________

Standard: ____________________

Age: Years: Sex: M/F

Weight: ________ kg, Height: ________ cm Chest: ________ cm Expansion: ________ cm

General health and nutritional state: ____________________

Protective inoculations: TAB/vaccination

Physical defects/deformities: ____________________

CVS ____________________

Respiratory system: ____________________

GI system Teeth: ____________________

Gums: ____________________

Liver: ____________________

Spleen: ____________________

CNS ____________________

Eyes/vision RE: ____________________ LE: ____________________

Ears/hearing RE: ____________________ LE: ____________________

Special points

____________________

____________________

____________________

____________________

____________________

____________________

**School class teaching program**

Deliver a class to school: ____________________

Topic: ____________________

Group: ____________________

Size of group: ____________________

Date: ____________________ Time: ____________________

Previous knowledge: ____________________

Method of teaching: ____________________

**General objectives:**

**Discuss about the topic:**

**Importance of—**

a. Personal hygiene

b. Environmental hygiene

c. Nutrition

d. Exercise

e. School report

- Introduction

- Geographical area

- Education level

- Staffs of primary school

- Functions of primary school

- Report of primary school

**Signature of Medical Officer/Principal**

# 13. HOME VISIT

The home visit is one of the most important aspects of community health services. Besides the healthy and the vulnerable population the vast majority of sick people are in their homes. Health service in the home requires technical skills, knowledge of preventive and therapeutic measures, teaching ability, judgment, and a full understanding of human relation.

## PURPOSES OF HOME VISITS

- In response to a need felt by an individual in the family as in case of sickness, delivery, surgery;
- As a part of a planned visiting program, e.g. routine prenatal visits;
- To investigate the source of an infectious disease in which case you may be rejected instead of being wanted;
- To follow through on some problem identified in the health center, school, industry or hospital;
- To assess nutritional and immunization status, environmental hazards and give health education;
- To follow treatment and care given by family members;
- To supervise and guide other health workers.

## PRINCIPLES OF WORKS

- Plan the work so that visits are made on the basis of need; divide your intensive area into units of 800 to 1,000 population each and plan for regular visits to the homes in selected units at a time;
- Be sensitive to the person's feelings and needs at the time of the visit;
- Understand the other person's point of view;
- Be sure of the scientific soundness of the subjects you discuss;
- Use safe technical skills, including hand-washing, inspection, etc.;
- Have a full understanding of your agency's policies;
- Attain a working knowledge of the community resources and use them wisely;
- Collect facts about the home, the patient and the environment and make an objective analysis of the facts as an initial step in visiting the home;
- Work with the person and family—plan jointly;
- Evaluate your own-quality is more important than quantity;
- Make a note of important facts in your diary;
- On return, record facts in the family folder and/or individual health cards.

## ADVANTAGES OF HOME VISIT

- The home visit permits the nurse to see the home and family situation in action.
- Family members will be more relaxed in their own surroundings.
- The home visit permits more realistic teaching in the actual situation, since socioeconomic background becomes clear.
- Family practices can be observed to form a basis for teaching.
- Other members of the family can be contacted who may have greater influence and control on member under nursing care.
- The family gains confidence in this direct personalized contact and are then free to raise questions and straighten the problems.
- The nurse has an opportunity to observe actual care given by family members.
- The home visit provides an opportunity to look for new health problem.

## STEPS IN HOME VISIT

### Fact Finding

The first step during a home visit is to study the clinical and other records to get an understanding of what has been done. This should give a lead to present needs and the community health nurse will be able to build on what has been done.

- Introduce yourself. Establish a friendly relationship through courtesy, graciousness and genuine interest.
- Observe inside and outside of the home of discern good and bad factors that may influence the situation.
- Talk with the person or persons concerned to find out what they know and understand about the situation. Use simple language.
- Discuss what has been done and what the person wants to do about the problem now and what plans he may have for the future.
- The condition pertaining to the environment and maternal and child health are the specific areas, which provide basic data for planning and giving appropriate nursing care and services.

### Examination and Analysis of the Facts

When the facts have been collected, the process of examining and analyzing begins. It is important to remember that true, honest, analysis is based on fact and not on opinion. The personal, environmental and economic factors, the emotional involvements and the spiritual aspects taken together constitute the usual health problem.

### Planning Action with the Individual or Family

Planning action with the person and family is of the greatest importance in all your work and relationship. Development from this point depends on your own attitude and ability to see the resource within the individual and family themselves.

### Action

What you do depend on the first three steps in the visit. Even though you enter the home with a definite idea and plan of what you will do, based on the information obtained in the health center, school, industry or other source.

### Follow-Through

It is one of the most important steps in the home visit. Follow-through on the patient mentioned involves assistance with hospital clearance; another visit just before she is admitted to help her understand hospital living.

## Use of Expert Technical Skill

Every professional worker needs tools and special skills. A nursing bag provides the nurse with the tools she needs to detect early signs and symptoms of disease, so that her report to the physician will be correct and intelligent.

## Evaluation of Service

Review each family record periodically; the results are not always immediately obvious. It takes months and sometimes years to see accomplishments.

# ASSIGNMENT–31 (A): FAMILY FOLDER

**I. Health Center**

Opened on date : ______________________

Name of the head of family : ______________________

Closed on date : ______________________

Religion/caste : ______________________

Village : ______________________

**1. Family Composition**

House No. : ______________________

a. Size of family : ______________________

Address : ______________________

b. Joint/single : ______________________

**Family History**

**Number of family members**

| Sl. No. | Name | Sex | Age | Relation to head of the family | Education | Occupation | Income per month | Immunization Status/ Health Status |
|---|---|---|---|---|---|---|---|---|
| | | | | | | | | |

**II. Environment**

1. **Housing**
   - Rented/own
   - No. of rooms
   - Persons per living room.
   - Dampness : Yes/No
   - Floor : Kutcha/Pucca/Other (specify)
   - Walls : Mud/Brick/With plaster/Other (specify)
   - Roof : Thatched/Tiles/Sheets/Concrete/Other (specify)
   - Ventilation in living room: Good/Satisfactory/Poor
   - Kitchen : Separate/Not separate/Smoky/Smokeless
   - Cattleshed : Not required/None/Attached/Separate
   - Electricity : Yes/No

   Locality : Congested/Semicongested/Open
2. **Drinking water source**—Well/Hand pump/Tube well/Other (Specify)
3. **Excreta disposal**—Open field/Latrine/Other (Specify)
4. **Refuse disposal**—Indiscriminate/Dumping/Composting/Other (Specify)
5. **Insects and rodents:**

   Flies—absent/present in a large number/present in a small number

   Mosquitoes—absent/present in a small number/present in a large number

   Rodents—absent/present in small number/present in a large number
6. **Animals/pets owned** ____________________

**III. Family Diet**

| Diet consumed veg/ non-veg/mixed | Number of meals per day | Average/weekly/ration for whole family | Remark |
|---|---|---|---|
| Milk | ______ Liters | | |
| Eggs | ______ gm/kg | | |
| Meat/Fish | ______ gm/kg | | |
| Rice | ______ gm/kg | | |
| Cereals, wheat, maize, bajra | ______ gm/kg | | |
| Sugar/jaggery | ______ gm/kg | | |
| Fat/Oils | ______ gm/kg | | |
| Vegetables (Green leafy) | ______ gm/kg | | |
| | ______ gm/kg | | |

## Comments on Diet

______________________________________________________________________
______________________________________________________________________
______________________________________________________________________
______________________________________________________________________
______________________________________________________________________
______________________________________________________________________
______________________________________________________________________
______________________________________________________________________
______________________________________________________________________
______________________________________________________________________
______________________________________________________________________
______________________________________________________________________
______________________________________________________________________
______________________________________________________________________
______________________________________________________________________

**IV. Family Economics**

- Number of earning members ______________________
- Dependency ratio ______________________
- Total family income per month Rs. ________ per capita income per month ______________

**Per month expenditure on:**

a. Food ______________
b. Housing ______________
c. Education ______________
d. Recreation ______________
e. Medical care ______________
f. Other ______________

Total Rs. ______________ per month

Saving ______________

**V. Social Problems**

- Unemployment ________________
- Indebtedness ________________
- Unmarried ________________
- Chronic sickness ________________
- Old invalid dependents ________________
- Other (Specify) ________________

**VI. Utilization of Health Facility**

- PHC ________________
- Private practitioner ________________
- Home remedies ________________

**VII. Field Notes (If any)**

**VIII. Progress Report**

(Note any improvement in the family in environment family dietary of any other characteristics)

| Date | Environment | Family dietary | Other | Signature |
|---|---|---|---|---|
| | | | | |

## FAMILY DATA COLLECTION CARD

Name of the head of the household: __________

Folder No: __________

Address: __________

A copy of location of map of house: __________

**State Your Aim and Objectives:** __________

**Date of first visit:** __________

- **Give a brief description of the family in terms of your observation.**

- **Describe the internal and external surroundings of the house, state the health risks and hazard identified, list your advice given to the family.**

- **State anticipated health needs, health-related problems and your plan of actions.**

**I. Family Characteristics**

Type of family : Nuclear/Joint/Extended
Size of family : ______
Religion : ______
State of origin : ______
Duration of stay (here) : ______
Monthly income (Total) : ______
No. of persons earning : ______
Source of income : ______
Monthly occupation : ______
Economic trade : ______
Status : ______
Chief diet : ______
Staple food : ______
Hobbies/leisure activities : ______
Psychosocial reaction : ______

Animals owned

1. ______ 2. ______ 3. ______

Poultry owned

1. ______ 2. ______ 3. ______

Pets owned

1. ______ 2. ______

Property owned

1. ______
2. ______
3. ______
4. ______

**II. Housing Condition**

1. Types of house : Katcha/Pucca, Own/Rented
2. No. of rooms : Presence of varandah
3. Living space per head : Presence of courtyard
4. Source of light : Condition of courtyard
5. Source of water :
6. Ventilation : Adequate/inadequate
7. Kitchen condition : Separate/Yes/No
   Type : Chullah/Stove/Gas/Heater
   Fuel used : Coal/Wood/Electricity/Oil
   Storage of food :

8. Drainage system : Open/Close
9. Disposal of water :
10. Domestic :
11. Human :
12. Domestic animal :
    Shed : Inside/outside the house
    Domestic pets : Yes/No, specify
    Kitchen garden-present/absent
13. Presence of trees : Yes/No, specify
    Shrubs : Yes/No

Measures for vector control ____________________

Vector nuisance : 1. __________ 2. __________
3. __________ 4. __________

Safe/unsafe For human health

Play facilities : Available indoor/outdoor

List accidents hazards : 1. __________ 2. __________

**III. Vital Events**

| During past 12 months | M | F |
|---|---|---|
| No. of births<br>No. of deaths<br>No. of abortions<br>No. of accidents<br>No. of pregnancies<br>No. of crimes/thefts | | |

## Causes of Disease/Death

| Sl. No. | Age | Sex | Cause of episode | Health care |
|---|---|---|---|---|
| | | | | |
| | | | | |
| | | | | |
| | | | | |
| | | | | |
| | | | | |
| | | | | |
| | | | | |
| | | | | |
| | | | | |
| | | | | |
| | | | | |
| | | | | |
| | | | | |

| Sl. No. | Age | Sex | Cause of episode | Health care |
|---|---|---|---|---|
| | | | | |
| | | | | |
| | | | | |
| | | | | |
| | | | | |
| | | | | |
| | | | | |
| | | | | |
| | | | | |
| | | | | |
| | | | | |
| | | | | |
| | | | | |
| | | | | |
| | | | | |
| | | | | |
| | | | | |
| | | | | |
| | | | | |
| | | | | |
| | | | | |
| | | | | |
| | | | | |
| | | | | |

**Source of health care preferred**

Military hospital : ______________________

Private practitioners : ______________________

Civil hospital : ______________________

Self-care : ______________________

## GENERAL INFORMATION OF FAMILY MEMBERS

(Persons living in the household)

| Sl. No. | Name | Relation with head of the family | Age | Sex | Marital Status | Educational status | Occupation | Income | Present health status | Disability | Immunization | Health care taken | Remarks |
|---|---|---|---|---|---|---|---|---|---|---|---|---|---|
| | | | | | | | | | | | | | |

A. General description of the members of the family not living in the household:

B. Eligible couples identified in the family:

C. Eligible couple practices Family planning Yes No

If yes, specify

If no, state reason

### Role of Family Members

**Q. What are the assigned household tasks?**

**a. Adults**

**Male:** ______________________

______________________

______________________

**Female:** ______________________

______________________

______________________

______________________

**b. Children**

**Boys:** ______________________

______________________

______________________

**Girls:** ______________________

______________________

______________________

______________________

______________________

**Q. Relation of family members. How do they get along?**

- Husband and wife ______________________
- Father and children ______________________

- Mother and children ____________________
- Children and children ____________________

**Q. Decision making in the family. Who makes the decision?**

- Major decisions ____________ (For example, hospitalization, family planning)
- Minor decision ____________ (For example, errands to market, collection of rations)

## COMPREHENSIVE FAMILY HEALTHCARE STUDY

### Antenatal and Postnatal Record

Name of the mother: ____________ Age: ______ Religion: ____________

Husband's name: ____________ Age: ______ Occupation: ____________

Address: ____________________

____________________

Gravida: ________ Para: ________ Date of LMP: ________ EDD.: ________

## HISTORY OF PREVIOUS PREGNANCIES

| Sl. No. | Age | Sex | FT/PM | Born alive/ stillborn | Living/ dead | Healthy otherwise | Abortion in month | Pregnancy/ NA | Labor/NA | Puerperium /NA |
|---|---|---|---|---|---|---|---|---|---|---|
| | | | | | | | | | | |

**Present Pregnancy**

| Date | Height of uterus | Position presentation | Head fixed/ floating | FHR/ meter | Weight | Urine | | BP | Hb | Investigations |
|---|---|---|---|---|---|---|---|---|---|---|
| | | | | | | Albumin | Sugar | | | |
| | | | | | | | | | | Blood VDRL general examinaion |
| | | | | | | | | | | Height |
| | | | | | | | | | | Nutrition |
| | | | | | | | | | | Heart |
| | | | | | | | | | | Lungs |
| | | | | | | | | | | Breasts |
| | | | | | | | | | | Abdomen |
| | | | | | | | | | | Anemia |
| | | | | | | | | | | Edema |
| | | | | | | | | | | Vaginal discharge |
| | | | | | | | | | | Other abnormalities |

| Date | Treatment | Health teaching | Remarks | Signature |
|---|---|---|---|---|
| | | | | |

## Internal

| Labor | Time | | | |
|---|---|---|---|---|
| | Date | Hours | Minutes | |
| Onset<br>Rupture of membranes<br>Birth of the child<br>placenta<br>Total hours<br>Nature of delivery | | | | Membranes and placenta<br>Hemorrhage<br>Perineum—intact/lacerated<br>Episiotomy<br>Infant<br>Sex<br>Wt<br>Length<br>Head circumference<br>Condition at birth |

## Progress of the Mother—Postnatal

| Date | Temperature | Pulse | Respiration | Height of uterus | Breasts | General condition and advice | Signature |
|---|---|---|---|---|---|---|---|
| | | | | | | | |

## Progress of the Child

| Date | Progress of the child | Signature |
|---|---|---|
| | | |

## Comprehensive Family Health Care Study
## Infant and Child Health Record

Name: ____________________
Sex: ____________________
Age physical exam: ____________________

### If Normal, Mark 'O'; and if Abnormal, Mark 'X'

- Father's name: ____________________
- Mother's name: ____________________
- Address: ____________________
- Date of birth: __________ Birth weight: __________
- Birth history: __________ Normal/abnormal __________
- Birth attendant: ____________________

| Month and year | Weight (kg) | Height (cm) | Month (and year) | Weight (kg) | Height (cm) |
|---|---|---|---|---|---|
| Jan.<br>Feb.<br>March<br>April<br>May<br>June | | | July<br>Aug<br>Sep<br>Oct<br>Nov<br>Dec | | |

**Immunizations**

| Name of vaccine | Date of immunization | | | | |
|---|---|---|---|---|---|
| BCG<br>DPT<br>TAB<br>Polio<br>TT<br>Cholera | | | | | |

**Development**

| | Yes | No |
|---|---|---|
| Head raised<br>Rolls over<br>Eruption of tooth<br>Sat with support<br>Without support<br>Sat alone walked with support<br>Talked<br>Walked alone<br>Bladder control<br>Bowel control | | |

| Physical exam | If Normal, Mark 'O'; If Abnormal Mark 'X' |
|---|---|
| Date<br>Age<br>Skin<br>Ears<br>Nose<br>Throat<br>Teeth and gum<br>Eyes<br>Bones<br>Joints<br>Liver<br>Spleen<br>Hb% | |
| **Dietery habits** | **Laboratory investigation** |
| | |

**Signs of Malnutrition (if observed, mark)**

- Xerosis
- Bitot's spot
- Keratomalacia
- Dermatitis
- Glossitis
- Angular stomatitis
- Bow legs
- Edema
- Others (specify)

## Infectious Diseases

| | Age | Yes | No | Others (specify) | Age | Yes | No |
|---|---|---|---|---|---|---|---|
| Primary complex<br>Chicken pox<br>Measles<br>Whooping cough<br>Mumps | | | | | | | |

| Date | General health: Nutritional status, development and illness if any | Nurses observation, treatment and health teaching | Sign of CH nurse |
|---|---|---|---|
| | | | |

## SCHOOL HEALTH SERVICE
### Medical History Sheet

Name of school: ______________________________

Name of pupil: ______________________________

Standard: ______________________________

______________________________

______________________________

Age: Years: Sex: M/F

Weight ________ kgs Height: ________ cms: Chest ________ cms: Expansion ________ cms:

General health and nutritional state: ______________________________

Protective inoculations: tab/vaccination: ______________________________

Physical defects/deformities ______________________________

CVS: ______________________________

Respiratory system: ______________________________

GI System Teeth ______________________________

Gums ______________________________

Liver ______________________________

Spleen ______________________________

CNS ______________________________

Eyes

Vision RE ______________________________

LE ______________________________

Ears

Hearing RE ______________________________

Special points LE ______________________________

______________________________

______________________________

______________________________

______________________________

______________________________

______________________________

**Signature of Medical Officer/Principal**

## ADULTS HEALTH CARD

Name of head of family: ____________________

House No: ____________________

Village: ____________ Sex ________ Year of birth ____________

Name: ____________________

Marital status: ____________________

Education: ____________________

Occupation: ____________________

____________________

____________________

Income: ____________________

| Immunization date | Habits | | Post illness | |
|---|---|---|---|---|
| BCG | Betel leaves | ( ) | Tuberculosis | ( ) |
| TT | Tobacco | ( ) | STD | ( ) |
| TAB | Smoking | ( ) | Malaria | ( ) |
| Cholera | Alcohols | ( ) | Filaria | ( ) |
| Others | Others (specify) | ( ) | Dysentry | ( ) |

### Laboratory Investigations

| Date | Specimen findings | Treatment | Signature |
|---|---|---|---|
| | | | |

## Morbidity

| Date | Complaints | Positive findings | Diagnosis | Treatment | Advice follow up | Signature |
|---|---|---|---|---|---|---|
| | | | | | | |

## Physical Health Assessment

Height: __________ cms General health and Eyes vision LE RE

Weight: __________ kg Nutritional status Ears hearing LE RE

Resp. system: Temp. P R

CNS:

Per abdomen: Liver: __________ Spleen: __________

Bowels and bladder function: Muscle skeletal system: Gait:

Mental and social health :

Adjustment aspects :

Family/work :

General outlook :

Hobbies interests :

Social circle :

Apparent physical/psychological defects

Special points:

# ASSIGNMENT–31 (B): FAMILY FOLDER

**I. Health Center**

Opened on date : ____________________

Name of the head of family : ____________________

Closed on date : ____________________

Religion/caste : ____________________

Village : ____________________

**Family composition**

House no. : ____________________

a. Size of family : ____________________

Address : ____________________

b. Joint/single : ____________________

____________________

## Family History

**Number of family members**

| Sl. No. | Name | Sex | Age | Relation to head of the family | Education | Occupation | Income per month | Immunization status/health status |
|---|---|---|---|---|---|---|---|---|
| | | | | | | | | |

**II. Environment**

**1. Housing**

- Rented/own
- No. of rooms
- Persons per living room
- Dampness : Yes/No
- Floor : Kutcha/Pucca, Other (Specify)
- Walls : Mud/Brick/With plaster/Other (Specify)
- Roof : Thatched/Tiles/Sheets/Concrete/Other (Specify)
- Ventilation in living room : Good/Satisfactory/Poor
- Kitchen : Separate/Not separate/Smoky/Smokeless
- Cattleshed : Not required/None/Attached/Separate
- Electricity : Yes/No
- Locality : Congested/Semicongested/Open

2. **Drinking water source** – Well/hand pump/tube well/other (specify)
3. **Excreta disposal** – Open field/latrine/other (specify)
4. **Refuse disposal** – Indiscriminate/dumping/composting/other (specify)
5. **Insects and rodents:**

   Flies – Absent/present in a large number/present in a small number

   Mosquitoes absent/present in a small number/present in a large number

   Rodents – absent/present in small number/present in a large numbers
6. **Animals/pets owned** ____________________

### III. Family Diet

| Diet consumed veg/ non-veg/mixed | Number of meals per day | Average/weekly/ration for whole family | Remark |
|---|---|---|---|
| Milk<br>Eggs<br>Meat/fish<br>Rice<br>Cereals wheat, maize, bajra<br>Sugar/jaggery<br>Fat/oils<br>Vegetables<br>Green leafy vegetables | ______ Liters<br>______ gm/kg<br>______ gm/kg<br>______ gm/kg<br>______ gm/kg<br>______ gm/kg<br>______ gm/kg<br>______ gm/kg | | |

## Comments on Diet

**IV. Family Economics**

- Number of earning members ______
- Dependency ratio ______
- Total family income per month Rs. ______ per capita income per month ______

**Per month expenditure on:**

a. Food ______
b. Housing ______
c. Education ______
d. Recreation ______
e. Medical care ______
f. Other ______

Total Rs. ______ per month
Saving ______

**V. Social problems**

- Unemployment ______
- Indebtedness ______
- Unmarried ______
- Chronic sickness ______
- Old invalid dependents ______
- Other (specify) ______

**VI. Utilization of health facility**

- PHC ______
- Private practitioner ______
- Home remedies ______

**VII. Field notes (If any)**

______

**VIII. Progress Report**

(Note any improvement in the family in environment family dietary of any other characteristics)

| Date | Environment | Family dietary | Other | Signature |
|---|---|---|---|---|
| | | | | |

## FAMILY DATA COLLECTION CARD

Name of the head of the household : ______

Folder no. : ______

Address : ______

______

A copy of location of map of house : ______

**State your aim and objectives:** ______

______

______

______

______

______

______

______

**Date of first visit:** ______

______

- **Give a brief description of the family in terms of your observation.**

______

______

______

______

______

______

- **Describe the internal and external surroundings of the house, state the health risks and hazard identified, list your advice given to the family.**

______

______

______

______

______

- **State anticipated health needs, health-related problems and your plan of actions.**

______

______

______

______

______

______

______

**I. Family Characteristics**

Type of family : Nuclear/joint/extended

Size of family : __________

Religion : __________

State of origin : __________

Duration of stay (here) : __________

Monthly income (total) : __________

No. of persons earning : __________

Source of income : __________

Monthly occupation : __________

Economic trade : __________

Status : __________

Chief diet : __________

Staple food : __________

Hobbies/leisure activities : __________

Psychosocial reaction: __________

Animals owned

1. ________ 2. ________ 3. ________

Poultry owned

1. ________ 2. ________ 3. ________

Pets owned

1. ________ 2. ________

Property owned

1. __________
2. __________
3. __________
4. __________

**II. Housing Condition**

1. Types of house : Katcha/Pucca, Own/Rented
2. No. of rooms : Presence of verandah
3. Living space per head : Presence of courtyard
4. Source of light : Condition of courtyard
5. Source of water :
6. Ventilation : Adequate/inadequate
7. Kitchen condition : Separate/yes/no
   Type : Chullah/Stove/Gas/Heater
   Fuel used : Coal/Wood/Electricity/Oil
   Storage of food :
8. Drainage system : Open/close
9. Disposal of water :
10. Domestic :
11. Human :
12. Domestic animal :
13. Shed : Inside/outside the house
14. Domestic pets : Yes/no, specify: Kitchen garden-present/absent
15. Presence of trees : Yes/no, specify
    Shrubs : Yes/no

Measures for vector control ____________________

Vector nuisance : 1. ____________ 2. ____________
3. ____________ 4. ____________

Safe/unsafe : For human health

Play facilities : Available indoor/outdoor

List accidents hazards : 1. ____________ 2. ____________

**III. Vital Events**

| During past 12 months | M | F |
|---|---|---|
| No. of births | | |
| No. of deaths | | |
| No. of abortions | | |
| No. of accidents | | |
| No. of pregnancies | | |
| No. of crimes/theft | | |

## Causes of Disease/death

| Sl. No. | Age | Sex | Cause of episode | Health care |
|---|---|---|---|---|
| | | | | |
| | | | | |
| | | | | |
| | | | | |
| | | | | |
| | | | | |
| | | | | |
| | | | | |
| | | | | |
| | | | | |
| | | | | |
| | | | | |
| | | | | |
| | | | | |
| | | | | |
| | | | | |
| | | | | |
| | | | | |
| | | | | |
| | | | | |
| | | | | |
| | | | | |
| | | | | |
| | | | | |
| | | | | |
| | | | | |
| | | | | |
| | | | | |
| | | | | |
| | | | | |
| | | | | |

**Source of health care preferred** : ______________________________

Military hospital : ______________________________

Private practitioners : ______________________________

Civil hospital : ______________________________

Self-care : ______________________________

## GENERAL INFORMATION OF FAMILY MEMBERS

(Persons Living in the Household)

| Sl. No. | Name | Relation with head of the family | Age | Sex | Martial | Status | Educa-tional status | Occupa-tion | Income | Present health status | Disabil-ity | Immuni-zation | Health care taken | Re-marks |
|---|---|---|---|---|---|---|---|---|---|---|---|---|---|---|
| | | | | | | | | | | | | | | |

A. General description of the members of the family not living in the household:

B. Eligible couples identified in the family:

C. Eligible couple practices Family planning Yes No

D. If yes, specify

E. If no, state reason

### Roles of Family Members

**Q. What are the assigned household tasks?**

a. **Adults**

**Male** ______________________________

______________________________

**Female**______________________________

______________________________

______________________________

______________________________

______________________________

b. **Children**

**Boys** ______________________________

______________________________

______________________________

**Girls** ______________________________

______________________________

______________________________

**Q. Relation of family members. How do they get along?**

- Husband and wife ______________________________
- Father and children ______________________________
- Mother and children ______________________________
- Children and children ______________________________

**Q. Decision making in the family. Who makes the decision?**

- Major decisions ________________ (For example, hospitalization, family planning)
- Minor decision ________________ (For example, errands to market, collection of rations)

## COMPREHENSIVE FAMILY HEALTH CARE STUDY

### Antenatal and Postnatal Record

Name of the mother: ________________ Age: ________ Religion: ________

Husband's name: ________________ Age: ________ Occupation: ________

Address: ________________________________

________________________________

________________________________

Gravida: ________ Para: ________ Date of LMP: ________ EDD: ________

### History of Previous Pregnancies

| Sl. No. | Age | Sex | FT/PM | Born alive/ still-born | Living/ dead | Healthy otherwise | Abortion in month | Pregnancy/NA | Labor/NA | Puerperium/ NA |
|---|---|---|---|---|---|---|---|---|---|---|
| | | | | | | | | | | |

**Present Pregnancy**

| Date | Height of uterus | Position presentation | Head fixed/ floating | FHR/ mt | Weight | Urine | | BP | HB | Investigations |
|---|---|---|---|---|---|---|---|---|---|---|
| | | | | | | Albumin | Sugar | | | |
| | | | | | | | | | | Blood VDRL general examinaion |
| | | | | | | | | | | Height |
| | | | | | | | | | | Nutrition |
| | | | | | | | | | | Heart |
| | | | | | | | | | | Lungs |
| | | | | | | | | | | Breasts |
| | | | | | | | | | | Abdomen |
| | | | | | | | | | | Anemia |
| | | | | | | | | | | Edema |
| | | | | | | | | | | Vaginal discharge |
| | | | | | | | | | | Other abnormalities |

| Date | Treatment | Health teaching | Remarks | Signature |
| --- | --- | --- | --- | --- |
| | | | | |

| Internal | | | | |
|---|---|---|---|---|
| Labor | Time | | | |
| | Date | Hour | Minute | |
| Onset<br>Rupture of membranes<br>Birth of the child<br>Placenta<br>Total hours<br>Nature of delivery | | | | Membranes and placenta<br>Hemorrhage<br>Perineum-Intact/Lacerated<br>Episiotomy<br>Infant<br>Sex<br>Weight<br>Length<br>Head circumference<br>Condition at birth |

## Progress of the Mother—Postnatal

| Date | Temp | Pulse | Resp | Height of uterus | Breasts | General condition and advice | Signature |
|---|---|---|---|---|---|---|---|
| | | | | | | | |

## Progress of the Child

| Date | Progress of the child | Signature |
|---|---|---|
| | | |

## Comprehensive Family Health Care Study
## Infant and Child Health Record

Name: ____________________

Sex: ____________________

Age____________________

Physical exam: ____________________

### If Normal, Mark 'O'; and If Abnormal, Mark 'X'

- Father's name: ____________________
- Mother's name: ____________________
- Address: ____________________
- Date of birth: ____________________ Birth weight: ____________________
- Birth history: ____________________ Normal/abnormal
- Birth attendant: ____________________

| Month and year | Weight (kg) | Height (cm) | Month (and year) | Weight (kg) | Height (cm) |
|---|---|---|---|---|---|
| Jan. | | | July | | |
| Feb. | | | Aug | | |
| March | | | Sep | | |
| April | | | Oct | | |
| May | | | Nov | | |
| June | | | Dec | | |

**Immunizations**

| Name of vaccine | Date of immunization | | | | |
|---|---|---|---|---|---|
| BCG | | | | | |
| DPT | | | | | |
| TAB | | | | | |
| Polio | | | | | |
| TT | | | | | |
| Cholera | | | | | |

**Development**

| | Yes | No |
|---|---|---|
| Head raised | | |
| Rolls over | | |
| Eruption of tooth | | |
| Sat with support | | |
| Without support | | |
| Sat alone walked with support | | |
| Talked | | |
| Walked alone | | |
| Bladder control | | |
| Bowel control | | |

| Physical exam | If normal mark 'o'; if abnormal, mark 'x' |
|---|---|
| Date<br>Age<br>Skin<br>Ears<br>Nose<br>Throat<br>Teeth and gum<br>Eyes<br>Bones<br>Joints<br>Liver<br>Spleen<br>Hb% | |
| **Dietery habits** | **Laboratory investigation** |
| | |

**Signs of Malnutrition (if observed, mark)**

- Xerosis
- Bitot's spot
- Keratomalacia
- Dermatitis
- Glossitis
- Angular stomatitis
- Bow legs
- Edema
- Others (specify)

## Infectious Diseases

| | Age | Yes | No | Others (specify) | Age | Yes | No |
|---|---|---|---|---|---|---|---|
| Primary complex<br>Chicken pox<br>Measles<br>Whooping cough<br>Mumps | | | | | | | |

| Date | General health: Nutritional status, development and illness if any | Nurses observation, treatment and health teaching | Sign of CH nurse |
|---|---|---|---|
| | | | |

## SCHOOL HEALTH SERVICE
### Medical History Sheet

Name of school: ______________________________

Name of pupil: ______________________________

Standard ______________________________

______________________________

______________________________

Age: __________ Years: Sex: M/F

Weight: ________ kg, Height __________ cm Chest ________ cm Expansion ________ cms

General health and nutritional state ______________________________

______________________________

Protective inoculations : TAB/vaccination

Physical defects/deformities: ______________________________

CVS ______________________________

Respiratory system ______________________________

Gi system Teeth ______________________________

Gums ______________________________

Liver ______________________________

Spleen ______________________________

CNS ______________________________

Eyes

Vision RE ______________________________

LE ______________________________

Ears RE ______________________________

Hearing LE ______________________________

Special points ______________________________

______________________________

______________________________

______________________________

______________________________

**Signature of Medical Officer/Principal**

## ADULTS HEALTH CARD

Special points: ______________________________

Name of head of family: ______________________________

House No.: ______________________________

Village: ______________ Sex __________ Year of birth ______________

Name: ______________________________

Marital status: ______________________________

Education: ______________________________

Occupation: ______________________________

______________________________

______________________________

Income: ______________________________

| Immunization date | Habits | Post illness |
|---|---|---|
| BCG<br>TT<br>TAB<br>Cholera<br>Others | Betel leaves ( )<br>Tobacco ( )<br>Smoking ( )<br>Alcohols ( )<br>Others (specify) ( ) | Tuberculosis ( )<br>STD ( )<br>Malaria ( )<br>Filaria ( )<br>Dysentry ( ) |

### Laboratory Investigations

| Date | Specimen findings | Treatment | Signature |
|---|---|---|---|
| | | | |

## Morbidity

| Date | Complaints | Positive findings | Diagnosis | Treatment | Advice follow-up | Signature |
|---|---|---|---|---|---|---|
| | | | | | | |

## Physical Health Assessment

Height ________ cm General health and Eyes vision LE RE

Weight ________ kg Nutritional status Ears hearing LE RE

Resp. system: Temp. P R

CNS :

Per abdomen: Liver: ________ Spleen: ________

Bowels and bladder function: Muscle skeletal system: Gait:

Mental and social health :

Adjustment aspects :

Family/work :

General outlook :

Hobbies/interests :

Social circle :

Apparent physical/psychological defects

Special points:

## ASSIGNMENT–31(C): FAMILY FOLDER

I. **Health center** : ______

Opened on date : ______

Name of the head of family : ______

Closed on date : ______

Religion/caste : ______

Village : ______

______

**Family composition** ______

House No. ______

a. Size of family : ______

Address : ______

______

b. Joint/single : ______

______

### Family History

**Number of Family Members**

| Sl. No. | Name | Sex | Age | Relation to head of the family | Education | Occupation | Income per month | Immunization status/health status |
|---|---|---|---|---|---|---|---|---|
| | | | | | | | | |

**II. Environment**

1. **Housing**
   - Rented/own
   - No. of rooms
   - Persons per living room
   - Dampness : Yes/No
   - Floor : Kutcha/Pucca/Other (Specify)
   - Walls : Mud/Brick/With Plaster/Other (Specify)
   - Roof : Thatched/Tiles/Sheets/Concrete/Other (Specify)
   - Ventilation in living room : Good/Satisfactory/Poor
   - Kitchen : Separate/Not separate/Smoky/Smokeless
   - Cattleshed : Not required/None/Attached/Separate
   - Electricity : Yes/No
   - Locality : Congested/Semi-congested/Open
2. **Drinking water source** – Well/Hand pump/Tube well/Other (Specify)
3. **Excreta disposal** – Open field/Latrine/Other (Specify)
4. **Refuse disposal** – Indiscriminate/Dumping/Composting/Other (Specify)
5. **Insects and rodents:**

   Flies—absent/present in a large number/present in a small number

   Mosquitoes—absence/present in a small number/present in a large number

   Rodents—absent/present in a small number/present in a large number
6. **Animals/Pets owned** ________________________________________

**III. Family Diet**

| Diet consumed veg/non-veg/mixed | Number of meals per day | Average/weekly/ration for whole family | Remark |
|---|---|---|---|
| Milk | ______ Liters | | |
| Eggs | ______ gm/kg | | |
| Meat/fish | ______ gm/kg | | |
| Rice | ______ gm/kg | | |
| Cereals wheat, maize, bajra | ______ gm/kg | | |
| Sugar/jaggery | ______ gm/kg | | |
| Fat/oils | ______ gm/kg | | |
| Vegetables | ______ gm/kg | | |
| Green leafy vegetables | | | |

## Comments on Diet

______________________________________________
______________________________________________
______________________________________________
______________________________________________
______________________________________________
______________________________________________
______________________________________________
______________________________________________
______________________________________________
______________________________________________
______________________________________________
______________________________________________
______________________________________________
______________________________________________

**IV. Family Economics**

- Number of earning members ______________________
- Dependency ratio ______________________
- Total family income per month Rs. ______________ per capita income per month ______________

**Per month expenditure on:**

a. Food ______________________
b. Housing ______________________
c. Education ______________________
d. Recreation ______________________
e. Medical care ______________________
f. Other ______________________

Total Rs. ______________________ per month
Saving ______________________

**V. Social problems**

- Unemployment ______
- Indebtedness ______
- Unmarried ______
- Chronic sickness ______
- Old invalid dependents ______
- Other (specify) ______

**VI. Utilization of Health Facility**

- PHC ______
- Private practitioner ______
- Home remedies ______

**VII. Field Notes (If any)**

**VIII. Progress Report**

(Note any improvement in the family in environment family dietary of any other characteristics)

| Date | Environment | Family dietary | Other | Signature |
|---|---|---|---|---|
| | | | | |

## FAMILY DATA COLLECTION CARD

Name of the head of the household : ____________________

Folder No. : ____________________

Address : ____________________

____________________

A copy of location of map of house : ____________________

**State your aim and objectives:** ____________________

**Date of 1st visit:** ____________________

- **Give a brief description of the family in terms of your observation.**

- **Describe the internal and external surroundings of the house, state the health risks and hazard identified, list your advice given to the family.**

- **State anticipated health needs, health-related problems and your plan of actions.**

**I. Family Characteristics**

Type of family : Nuclear/Joint/Extended

Size of family : ______________________

Religion : ______________________

State of origin : ______________________

Duration of stay (here) : ______________________

Monthly income (total) : ______________________

No. of persons earning : ______________________

Source of income : ______________________

Monthly occupation : ______________________

Economic trade : ______________________

Status : ______________________

Chief diet : ______________________

Staple food : ______________________

Hobbies/leisure activities : ______________________

Psychosocial reaction : ______________________

Animals owned

1. ____________ 2. ____________ 3. ____________

Poultry owned

1. ____________ 2. ____________ 3. ____________

Pets owned

1. ____________ 2. ____________

Property owned

1. ______________________
2. ______________________
3. ______________________
4. ______________________

**II. Housing Condition**

| | | |
|---|---|---|
| 1. | Types of house | : Katcha/Pucca, Own/Rented |
| 2. | No. of rooms | : Presence of verandah |
| 3. | Living space per head | : Presence of courtyard |
| 4. | Source of light | : Condition of courtyard |
| 5. | Source of water | : |
| 6. | Ventilation | : Adequate/inadequate |
| 7. | Kitchen condition | : Separate/Yes/No |
| 8. | Type | : Chullah/Stove/Gas/Heater |
| 9. | Fuel used | : Coal/Wood/Electricity/Oil |
| 10. | Storage of food | : |
| 11. | Drainage system | : Open/Close |
| 12. | Disposal of water | : |
| 13. | Domestic | : |
| 14. | Human | : |
| 15. | Domestic animal | : |
| 16. | Shed | : Inside/Outside the house |
| 17. | Domestic pets | : Yes/No, specify<br>Kitchen Garden, present/absent |
| 18. | Presence of trees | : Yes/No, specify |
| | Shrubs | : Yes/No |
| | Measures for vector control | |
| | Vector nuisance | : 1. ____________ 2. ____________<br>3. ____________ 4. ____________ |
| | Safe/unsafe | For human health |
| | Play facilities | : Available indoor/outdoor |
| | List accidents hazards | : 1. ____________ 2. ____________ |

**III. Vital Events**

| During past 12 months | M | F |
|---|---|---|
| No. of births | | |
| No. of deaths | | |
| No. of abortions | | |
| No. of accidents | | |
| No. of pregnancies | | |
| No. of crimes/theft | | |

## Causes of Disease/Death

| Sl. No. | Age | Sex | Cause of episode | Health care |
|---|---|---|---|---|
| | | | | |
| | | | | |
| | | | | |
| | | | | |
| | | | | |
| | | | | |
| | | | | |
| | | | | |
| | | | | |
| | | | | |
| | | | | |
| | | | | |
| | | | | |
| | | | | |
| | | | | |
| | | | | |
| | | | | |
| | | | | |
| | | | | |
| | | | | |
| | | | | |
| | | | | |
| | | | | |
| | | | | |
| | | | | |
| | | | | |
| | | | | |
| | | | | |
| | | | | |
| | | | | |
| | | | | |
| | | | | |
| | | | | |
| | | | | |
| | | | | |

**Source of health care preferred** : ______________________

Military hospital : ______________________

Private practitioners : ______________________

Civil hospital : ______________________

Self-care : ______________________

## GENERAL INFORMATION OF FAMILY MEMBERS

**(Persons Living in the House Hold)**

| Sl. No. | Name | Relation with head of the family | Age | Sex | Marital | Status | Educa-tional status | Occu-pation | Income | Present health status | Dis-ability | Immu-niza-tion | Health care taken | Re-marks |
|---|---|---|---|---|---|---|---|---|---|---|---|---|---|---|
| | | | | | | | | | | | | | | |

A. General description of the members of the family not living in the household:

B. Eligible couples identified in the family:

C. Eligible couple practices Family planning Yes No

D. If yes, specify

E. If no, state reason.

## Roles of Family Members

**Q. What are the assigned household tasks ?**

a. **Adults**

**Male:** ______________________

______________________

**Female:** ______________________

______________________

______________________

______________________

b. **Children:**

**Boys:** ______________________

______________________

______________________

______________________

**Girls:** ______________________

______________________

______________________

______________________

**Q. Relation of family members. How do they get along ?**

- Husband and wife ____________________
- Father and children ____________________
- Mother and children ____________________
- Children and children ____________________

**Q. Decision making in the family. Who makes the decision?**

- Major decisions ____________________ (for e.g. hospitalization, family planning)
- Minor decision ____________________ (for e.g. errands to market, collection of rations)

## COMPREHENSIVE FAMILY HEALTH CARE STUDY

### Antenatal and Postnatal Record

Name of the mother: ____________________ Age: __________ Religion: ____________________

Husband's name: ____________________ Age: __________ Occupation: ____________________

Address: ____________________

____________________

____________________

____________________

Gravida: __________ Para: __________ Date of LMP: __________ EDD: __________

### History of Previous Pregnancies

| Sl. No. | Age | Sex | FT/PM | Born alive/ still- born | Living/ dead | Healthy otherwise | Abortion in month | Pregnancy/NA | Labor/NA | Puerperium/ NA |
|---|---|---|---|---|---|---|---|---|---|---|
| | | | | | | | | | | |

**Present Pregnancy**

| Date | Height of uterus | Position presenta-tion | Head fixed/ floating | FHR/mt | Weight | Urine | | BP | Hb | Investigations |
|---|---|---|---|---|---|---|---|---|---|---|
| | | | | | | Albumin | Sugar | | | |
| | | | | | | | | | | Blood VDRL general exami-nation<br>Height<br>Nutrition<br>Heart<br>Lungs<br>Breasts<br>Abdomen<br>Anemia<br>Edema<br>Vaginal discharge<br>Other abnormalities |

| Date | Treatment | Health teaching | Remarks | Signature |
|---|---|---|---|---|
| | | | | |

| Internal | | | | | |
|---|---|---|---|---|---|
| Labor | Time | | | | |
| | Date | Hours | Minutes | | |
| Onset<br>Rupture of membranes<br>Birth of the child<br>Placenta<br>Total hours<br>Nature of delivery | | | | | Membranes and placenta<br>Hemorrhage<br>Perineum-Intact/Lacerated<br>Episiotomy<br>Infant<br>Sex<br>Weight<br>Length<br>Head circumference<br>Condition at birth |

## Progress of the Mother—Postnatal

| Date | Temp | Pulse | Resp | Height of uterus | Breasts | General condition and advice | Signature |
|---|---|---|---|---|---|---|---|
| | | | | | | | |

## Progress of the Child

| Date | Progress of the child | Signature |
|---|---|---|
| | | |

## Comprehensive Family Health Care Study
## Infant and Child Health Record

Name ____________________
Sex ____________________
Age ____________________
Physical Exam. ____________________

### If Normal, Mark 'O'; and If Abnormal, Mark 'X'

- Father's name: ____________________
- Mother's name: ____________________
- Address: ____________________
- Date of birth: __________ Birth weight: __________
- Birth history: ____________________ Normal/abnormal
- Birth attendant: ____________________

| Month and Year | Weight (kg) | Height (cm) | Month and Year | Weight (kg) | Height (cm) |
|---|---|---|---|---|---|
| Jan | | | July | | |
| Feb | | | Aug | | |
| March | | | Sep | | |
| April | | | Oct | | |
| May | | | Nov | | |
| June | | | Dec | | |

**Immunizations**

| Name of vaccine | Date of immunization | | | | |
|---|---|---|---|---|---|
| BCG | | | | | |
| DPT | | | | | |
| TAB | | | | | |
| Polio | | | | | |
| TT | | | | | |
| Cholera | | | | | |

**Development**

| | Yes | No |
|---|---|---|
| Head raised | | |
| Rolls over | | |
| Eruption of tooth | | |
| Sat with support | | |
| Without support | | |
| Sat alone walked with support | | |
| Talked | | |
| Walked alone | | |
| Bladder control | | |
| Bowel control | | |

| Physical exam | If normal, mark 'O'; if abnormal, mark 'X' |
|---|---|
| Date | |
| Age | |
| Skin | |
| Ears | |
| Nose | |
| Throat | |
| Teeth and Gum | |
| Eyes | |
| Bones | |
| Joints | |
| Liver | |
| Spleen | |
| Hb% | |
| **Dietery habits** | **Laboratory investigation** |
| | |

**Signs of Malnutrition (if observed, mark)**

- Xerosis
- Bitot's spot
- Keratomalacia
- Dermatitis
- Glossitis
- Angular stomatitis
- Bow legs
- Edema
- Others (specify)

## Infectious Diseases

| | Age | Yes | No | Others (specify) | Age | Yes | No |
|---|---|---|---|---|---|---|---|
| Primary complex<br>Chicken pox<br>Measles<br>Whooping cough<br>Mumps | | | | | | | |

| Date | General health: Nutritional status, development and illness, if any | Nurses observation, treatment and health teaching | Sign of CH nurse |
|---|---|---|---|
| | | | |

## SCHOOL HEALTH SERVICE

### Medical History Sheet

Name of school: ______________________________

Name of pupil: ______________________________

Standard ______________________________

______________________________

______________________________

Age: __________ Years Sex: M/F

Weight __________ Kgs, Hight __________ cms Chest __________ cms Expansion __________ cms

General health and nutritional state: ______________________________

______________________________

Protective inoculations: TAB/vaccination

Physical defects/deformities: ______________________________

CVS: ______________________________

Respiratory system ______________________________

GI system Teeth ______________________________

Gums ______________________________

Liver ______________________________

Spleen ______________________________

CNS ______________________________

Eyes ______________________________

Vision RE ______________________________

LE ______________________________

Ears RE ______________________________

Hearing LE ______________________________

Special points ______________________________

______________________________

______________________________

______________________________

______________________________

______________________________

**Signature of Medical Officer/Principal**

# ADULTS HEALTH CARD

Special Points: ___________________________

Name of head of family: ___________________________

House No.: ___________________________

Village: ___________________ Sex __________ Year of birth __________

Name: ___________________________

Marital status: ___________________________

Education: ___________________________

Occupation: ___________________________

___________________________

___________________________

Income: ___________________________

| Immunizations date | Habits | | Post illness | |
|---|---|---|---|---|
| BCG | Betel leaves | ( ) | Tuberculosis | ( ) |
| TT | Tobacco | ( ) | STD | ( ) |
| TAB | Smoking | ( ) | Malaria | ( ) |
| Cholera | Alcohols | ( ) | Filaria | ( ) |
| Others | Others (specify) | ( ) | Dysentry | ( ) |

## Laboratory Investigations

| Date | Specimen findings | Treatment | Signature |
|---|---|---|---|
| | | | |

## Morbidity

| Date | Complaints | Positive findings | Diagnosis | Treatment | Advice follow-up | Signature |
|---|---|---|---|---|---|---|
| | | | | | | |

## Physical Health Assessment

Height ______ cm. General health and Eyes vision LE RE

Weight kg. Nutritional status Ears hearing LE RE

Resp. system: Temp. P R

CNS:

Per abdomen: Liver: ______________ Spleen ______

Bowels and bladder function : Muscle skeletal system: Gait:

Mental and social health :

Adjustment aspects :

Family/work :

General outlook :

Hobbies interests :

Social circle : Apparent physical/psychological defects

Special points:

## ASSIGNMENT–31 (D): FAMILY FOLDER

I. **Health Center** : ____________________

Opened on date : ____________________

Name of the head of family : ____________________

Closed on date : ____________________

Religion/caste : ____________________

Village : ____________________

**Family composition**

House No. : ____________________

a. Size of family : ____________________

Address : ____________________

b. Joint/single : ____________________

**Family History**

**Number of Family Members**

| Sl. No. | Name | Sex | Age | Relation to head of the family | Education | Occupation | Income per month | Immunization status/health status |
|---|---|---|---|---|---|---|---|---|
| | | | | | | | | |

## II. Environment

1. **Housing**
   - Rented/own
   - No. of rooms
   - Persons per living room
   - Dampness : Yes/No
   - Floor : Kutcha/Pucca/Other (Specify)
   - Walls : Mud/Brick/With plaster/Other (Specify)
   - Roof : Thatched/Tiles/Sheets/Concrete/Other (Specify)
   - Ventilation in living room : Good/Satisfactory/Poor
   - Kitchen : Separate/Not separate/Smoky/Smokeless
   - Cattleshed : Not required/None/Attached/Separate
   - Electricity : Yes/No
   - Locality : Congested/Semicongested/Open
2. **Drinking Water Source** – Well/Hand pump/Tube well/Other (Specify)
3. **Excreta Disposal** – Open field/Latrine/Other (Specify)
4. **Refuse Disposal** – Indiscriminate/Dumping/Composting/Other (Specify)
5. **Insects and Rodents:**
   Flies–absent/present in a large number/present in a small number
   Mosquitoes–absent/present in small number/present in a large number
   Rodents–absent/present in a small number/present in a large number
6. **Animals/Pets Owned** ________________

### III. Family Diet

| Diet consumed veg/non-veg/mixed | Number of meals per day | Average/weekly/ration for whole family | Remark |
|---|---|---|---|
| Milk | ________ Liters | | |
| Eggs | ________ gm/kg | | |
| Meat/fish | ________ gm/kg | | |
| Rice | ________ gm/kg | | |
| Cereals wheat, maize, bajra | ________ gm/kg | | |
| Sugar/jaggery | ________ gm/kg | | |
| Fat/oils | ________ gm/kg | | |
| Vegetables | ________ gm/kg | | |
| Green leafy vegetables | | | |

**Comments on Diet**

___

___

___

___

___

___

___

___

___

___

___

**IV. Family Economics**

- Number of earning members ___
- Dependency ratio ___
- Total family income per month Rs. ___ per capita income per month ___

**Per month expenditure on:**

a. Food ___
b. Housing ___
c. Education ___
d. Recreation ___
e. Medical care ___
f. Other ___

Total Rs. ___ per month
Saving ___

**V. Social Problems**

- Unemployment ___
- Indebtedness ___
- Unmarried ___
- Chronic sickness ___
- Old invalid dependents ___
- Other (specify) ___

**VI. Utilization of Health Facility**

- PHC
- Private practitioner
- Home remedies

**VII. Field Notes (If any)**

___

___

___

___

___

___

**VIII. Progress Report**

(Note any improvement in the family in environment family dietary of any other characteristics)

| Date | Environment | Family dietary | Other | Signature |
|---|---|---|---|---|
| | | | | |

## FAMILY DATA COLLECTION CARD

Name of the head of the household : ______
Folder no. : ______
Address : ______

A copy of location of map of house : ______

**State your aim and objectives:** ______

**Date of 1st visit:** ______

- **Give a brief description of the family in terms of your observation.**

- **Describe the internal and external surroundings of the house, state the health risks and hazard identified, list your advice given to the family.**

- **State anticipated health needs, health-related problems and your plan of actions.**

**I. Family Characteristics**

Type of family : Nuclear/Joint/Extended
Size of family : __________
Religion : __________
State of origin : __________
Duration of stay (here) : __________
Monthly income (total) : __________
No. of persons earning : __________
Source of income : __________
Monthly occupation : __________
Economic trade : __________
Status : __________
Chief diet : __________
Staple food : __________
Hobbies/leisureactivities: __________
Psychosocial reaction : __________

Animals owned
1. __________ 2. __________ 3. __________

Poultry owned
1. __________ 2. __________ 3. __________

Pets owned
1. __________ 2. __________

Property owned
1. __________
2. __________
3. __________
4. __________

**II. Housing Condition**

1. Types of house : Katcha/Pucca, Own/rented
2. No. of rooms : Presenence of varandah
3. Living space per head Presence of courtyard
4. Source of light : Condition of courtyard
5. Source of water :
6. Ventilation : Adequate/inadequate
7. Kitchen condition : Separate/Yes/No
8. Type : Chullah/Stove/Gas/Heater
9. Fuel used : Coal/Wood/Electricity/Oil
10. Storage of food :
11. Drainage system : Open/Close

12. Disposal of water :
13. Domestic :
14. Human :
15. Domestic animal :
16. Shed : Inside/Outside the house
17. Domestic pets : Yes/No, specify (Kitchen Garden, present/absent)
18. Presence of trees : Yes/No, specify
    shrubs : Yes/No

Measures for vector control ____________

Vector Nuisance : 1. ____________ 2. ____________
3. ____________ 4. ____________

Safe/Unsafe For Human health

Play facilities : available indoor/outdoor

List accidents hazards : 1. ____________ 2. ____________

## III. VITAL EVENTS

| During past 12 months | M | F |
|---|---|---|
| No. of births<br>No. of deaths<br>No. of abortions<br>No. of accidents<br>No. of pregnancies<br>No. of crimes/thefts | | |

## Causes of Disease/Death

| Sl. No. | Age | Sex | Cause of episode | Health care |
|---|---|---|---|---|
| | | | | |
| | | | | |
| | | | | |
| | | | | |
| | | | | |
| | | | | |
| | | | | |
| | | | | |
| | | | | |
| | | | | |
| | | | | |
| | | | | |

*Contd...*

*Contd...*

| | | | | |
|---|---|---|---|---|
| | | | | |
| | | | | |
| | | | | |
| | | | | |
| | | | | |
| | | | | |
| | | | | |
| | | | | |
| | | | | |
| | | | | |
| | | | | |

**Source of health care preferred** : ______________________
Military hospital : ______________________
Private practitioners : ______________________
Civil hospital : ______________________
Self care : ______________________

## GENERAL INFORMATION OF FAMILY MEMBERS

### (Persons Living in the Household)

| Sl. No. | Name | Relation with head of the family | Age | Sex | Marital | Status | Educational status | Occupation | Income | Present health status | Disability | Immunization | Health care taken | Remarks |
|---|---|---|---|---|---|---|---|---|---|---|---|---|---|---|
| | | | | | | | | | | | | | | |

A. General description of the members of the family not living in the household:
B. Eligible couples identified in the family:
C. Eligible couple practices Family planning Yes No
D. If yes, specify
E. If no, state reason

## Roles of Family Members

**Q. What are the assigned household tasks ?**

a. **Adults**

**Male:** ____________________

____________________

**Female:** ____________________

____________________

____________________

____________________

____________________

____________________

b. **Children:**

**Boys:** ____________________

____________________

____________________

____________________

**Girls:** ____________________

____________________

____________________

____________________

**Q. Relation of family members. How do they get along ?**

- Husband and wife ____________________
- Father and children ____________________
- Mother and children ____________________
- Children and children ____________________

**Q. Decision making in the family. Who makes the decision ?**

- Major decisions ____________________ (For example, hospitalization, family planning)
- Minor decision ____________________ (For example, errands to market, collection of rations)

## COMPREHENSIVE FAMILY HEALTH CARE STUDY

### Antenatal and Postnatal Record

Name of the Mother: ____________________ Age: ________ Religion: ____________________

Husband's Name: ____________________ Age: ________ Occupation: ____________________

Address: ____________________

____________________

____________________

Gravida: ____________ Para: ____________ Date of LMP: ____________ EDD: ____________

## History of Previous Pregnancies

| Sl. No. | Age | Sex | FT/PM | Born alive/still-born | Living/ dead | Healthy oth-erwise | Abortion in month | Pregnancy/NA | Labor/NA | Puerperium/ NA |
|---|---|---|---|---|---|---|---|---|---|---|
| | | | | | | | | | | |

## Present Pregnancy

| Date | Height of uterus | Position presenta-tion | Head fixed/ floating | FHR/m | Weight | Urine | | BP | Hb | Investigations |
|---|---|---|---|---|---|---|---|---|---|---|
| | | | | | | Albumin | Sugar | | | |
| | | | | | | | | | | Blood VDRL |
| | | | | | | | | | | Height |
| | | | | | | | | | | Nutrition |
| | | | | | | | | | | Heart |
| | | | | | | | | | | Lungs |
| | | | | | | | | | | Breasts |
| | | | | | | | | | | Abdomen |
| | | | | | | | | | | Anemia |
| | | | | | | | | | | Edema |
| | | | | | | | | | | Vaginal discharge |
| | | | | | | | | | | Other abnormalities |

| Date | Treatment | Health teaching | Remarks | Signature |
|---|---|---|---|---|
| | | | | |

| Internal | | | | |
|---|---|---|---|---|
| Labor | Time | | | |
| | Date | Hours | Minutes | |
| Onset<br>Rupture of membranes<br>Birth of the child<br>Placenta<br>Total hours<br>Nature of delivery | | | | Membranes and placenta<br>Hemorrhage<br>Perineum-intact/lacerated<br>Episiotomy<br>Infant<br>Sex<br>Weight<br>Length<br>Head circumference<br>Condition at birth |

## Progress of the Mother—Postnatal

| Date | Temp | Pulse | Resp | Height of uterus | Breasts | General condition and advice | Signature |
|---|---|---|---|---|---|---|---|
| | | | | | | | |

## Progress of the Child

| Date | Progress of the child | Signature |
|---|---|---|
| | | |

## Comprehensive Family Health Care Study
## Infant and Child Health Record

Name : ____________________
Sex : ____________________
Age : ____________________
Physical Exam : ____________________

### If Normal, Mark 'O'; and If Abnormal, Mark 'X'

- Father's Name: ____________________
- Mother's Name: ____________________
- Address: ____________________
- Date of Birth: ____________________ Birth weight: ____________________
- Birth History: ____________________ Normal/Abnormal
- Birth Attendant: ____________________

| Month and Year | Weight (kg) | Height (cm) | Month and Year | Weight (kg) | Height (cm) |
|---|---|---|---|---|---|
| Jan<br>Feb<br>March<br>April<br>May<br>June | | | July<br>Aug<br>Sep<br>Oct<br>Nov<br>Dec | | |

**Immunizations**

| Name of vaccine | Date of Immunization | | | | |
|---|---|---|---|---|---|
| BCG<br>DPT<br>TAB<br>Polio<br>TT<br>Cholera | | | | | |

**Development**

| | Yes | No |
|---|---|---|
| Head raised<br>Rolls over<br>Eruption of tooth<br>Sat with support<br>Without support<br>Sat alone walked with support<br>Talked<br>Walked alone<br>Bladder control<br>Bowel control | | |

| Physical exam | If Normal, Mark 'O'; If Abnormal, Mark 'X' |
|---|---|
| Date<br>Age<br>Skin<br>Ears<br>Nose<br>Throat<br>Teeth and gum<br>Eyes<br>Bones<br>Joints<br>Liver<br>Spleen<br>Hb% | |
| **Dietery habits** | **Laboratory Investigation** |
| | |

**Signs of Malnutrition (if observed, mark)**

- Xerosis
- Bitot's spot
- Keratomalacia
- Dermatitis
- Glossitis
- Angular stomatitis
- Bow legs
- Edema
- Others (specify)

## Infectious Diseases

| | Age | Yes | No | Others (specify) | Age | Yes | No |
|---|---|---|---|---|---|---|---|
| Primary complex | | | | | | | |
| Chicken pox | | | | | | | |
| Measles | | | | | | | |
| Whooping cough | | | | | | | |
| Mumps | | | | | | | |

| Date | General health: Nutritional status, development and illness if any | Nurses observation, treatment and health teaching | Signature of CH nurse |
|---|---|---|---|
| | | | |

## School Health Service
## (Medical History Sheet)

Name of school: ____________________

Name of pupil: ____________________

Standard: ____________________

____________________

____________________

Age: ________ years Sex: M/F

Weight: ________ kg Hight: ________ cms. Chest: ________ cms. Expansion: ________ cms.

General health and nutritional state

Protective inoculations: TAB/vaccination

Physical defects/deformities: ____________________

CVS: ____________________

Respiratory system: ____________________

GI system Teeth: ____________________

Gums: ____________________

Live: ____________________

Spleen: ____________________

CNS: ____________________

Eyes

Vision RE: ____________________

LE: ____________________

Ears RE: ____________________

Hearing LE: ____________________

Special points: ____________________

____________________

____________________

____________________

____________________

**Signature of Medical Officer/Principal**

## Adults Health Card

Special points: ______

Name of head of family: ______

House No: ______

Village: ______ Sex: ______ Year of birth: ______

Name: ______

Marital status: ______

Education: ______

Occupation: ______

______

______

Income: ______

| Immunization date | Habits | Post illness |
|---|---|---|
| BCG | Betel leaves ( ) | Tuberculosis ( ) |
| TT | Tobacco ( ) | STD ( ) |
| TAB | Smoking ( ) | Malaria ( ) |
| Cholera | Alcohols ( ) | Filaria ( ) |
| Others | Others (specify) ( ) | Dysentry ( ) |

## Laboratory Investigations

| Date | Specimen findings | Treatment | Signature |
|---|---|---|---|
| | | | |

## Morbidity

| Date | Complaints | Positive findings | Diagnosis | Treatment | Advice follow up | Signature |
|---|---|---|---|---|---|---|
| | | | | | | |

## Physical Health Assessment

Height _____ cms General health and Eyes vision LE RE
Weight _____ kg nutritional status Ears hearing LE RE
Resp. system: Temp P R
CNS:
Per abdomen: Liver : __________ Spleen __________
Bowels and bladder function: Muscle skeletal system: Gait:
Mental and social health :
Adjustment aspects :
Family/Work :
General outlook :
Hobbies interests :
Social circle :

Apparent physical/psychological defects
Special points:

# ASSIGNMENT–31 (E): FAMILY FOLDER

I. Health center : ____________________
Opened on date : ____________________
Name of the head of family : ____________________
Closed on date : ____________________
Religion/caste : ____________________
Village : ____________________
**Family composition** : ____________________
House No. : ____________________
a. Size of family : ____________________
Address : ____________________
b. Joint/single : ____________________
____________________

## Family History

### Number of family members

| Sl. No. | Name | Sex | Age | Relation to head of the family | Education | Occupation | Income per month | Immunization status/ health status |
|---|---|---|---|---|---|---|---|---|
| | | | | | | | | |

**II. Environment**

1. **Housing**
   - Rented/own
   - No. of rooms
   - Persons per living room
   - Dampness : Yes/No
   - Floor : Katcha/Pucca, Other (specify)
   - Walls : Mud/Brick/with plaster/other (specify)
   - Roof : Thatched/tiles/sheets/concrete/other (specify)
   - Ventilation in living room – Good/satisfactory/poor
   - Kitchen : Separate/Not separate/Smoky/Smokeless
   - Cattleshed : Not required/None/Attached/Separate
   - Electricity : Yes/No; Locality – Congested/Semi-congested/Open

2. **Drinking water source** – Well/Hand pump/Tube well/Other (specify)
3. **Excreta disposal** – Open field/Latrine/Other (specify)
4. **Refuse disposal** – Indiscriminate/dumping/composting/other (specify)
5. **Insects and rodents:**
   Flies–absent/present in a large number/present in a small number
   Mosquitoes–absence/present in a small number/present in a large number
   Rodents–absent/present in a small number/present in a large number
6. **Animals/Pets Owned** ______________________________

**III. Family Diet**

| Diet consumed veg/non-veg/mixed | Number of meals per day | Average/weekly/ration for whole family | Remark |
|---|---|---|---|
| Milk | ________ Liters | | |
| Eggs | ________ gm/kg | | |
| Meat/Fish | ________ gm/kg | | |
| Rice | ________ gm/kg | | |
| Cereals wheat, maize, bajra | ________ gm/kg | | |
| Sugar/jaggery | ________ gm/kg | | |
| Fat/oils | ________ gm/kg | | |
| Vegetables | ________ gm/kg | | |
| Green leafy vegetables | | | |

## Comments on Diet

______________________________

**IV. Family Economics**

- Number of earning members __________
- Dependency ratio __________
- Total family income per month Rs. __________ per capita income per month __________

**Per month expenditure on:**

a: Food __________
b: Housing __________
c: Education __________
d: Recreation __________
e: Medical care __________
f: Other __________

Total Rs. __________ per month

Saving __________

**V. Social Problems**

- Unemployment __________
- Indebtedness __________
- Unmarried __________
- Chronic sickness __________
- Old invalid dependents __________
- Other (specify) __________

**VI. Utilization of Health Facility**

- PHC __________
- Private practitioner __________
- Home remedies __________

**VII. Field Notes (If any)**

**VIII. Progress Report**

(Note: Any improvement in the family in environment family dietary of any other characteristics)

| Date | Environment | Family dietary | Other | Signature |
|---|---|---|---|---|
| | | | | |

## FAMILY DATA COLLECTION CARD

Nameoftheheadofthehousehold: __________

Folder No: __________

Address: __________

A copy of location of map of house: __________

**State Your Aim and Objectives:** __________

**Date of 1st visit:** __________

- **Give a brief description of the family in terms of your observation:**

- **Describe the internal and external surroundings of the house, state the health risks and hazard identified, list your advice given to the family.**

- **State anticipated health needs, health-related problems and your plan of actions.**

**I. Family Characteristics**

Type of family : Nuclear/Joint/Extended
Size of family : ______
Religion : ______
State of origin : ______
Duration of stay (here) : ______
Monthly income (total) : ______
No. of persons earning : ______
Source of income : ______
Monthly occupation : ______
Economic trade : ______
Status : ______
Chief diet : ______
Staple food : ______
Hobbies/leisure activities: ______
Psychosocial reaction : ______

Animals owned

1. ______ 2. ______ 3. ______

Poultry owned

1. ______ 2. ______ 3. ______

Pets owned

1. ______ 2. ______

Property owned

1. ______
2. ______
3. ______
4. ______

**II. Housing Condition**

1. Types of house : Katcha/Pucca, Own/Rented
2. No. of rooms : Presenence of varandah
3. Living space per head Presence of courtyard
4. Source of light : Condition of courtyard
5. Source of water :
6. Ventilation : Adequate/inadequate
7. Kitchen condition : Separate/Yes/No
8. Type : Chullah/Stove/Gas/Heater
9. Fuel used : Coal/Wood/Electricity/Oil
10. Storage of food :
11. Drainage system : Open/Close
12. Disposal of water :
13. Domestic :
14. Human :
15. Domestic animal :
16. Shed : Inside/Outside the house
17. Domestic pets : Yes/No, specify: Kitchen Garden, present/absent
18. Presence of trees : Yes/No, specify
    Shrubs : Yes/No

Measures for vector control ____________________

Vector nuisance : 1. ____________ 2. ____________

3. ____________ 4. ____________

Safe/Unsafe For human health

Play facilities : Available indoor/outdoor

List accidents hazards : 1. ____________ 2. ____________

**III. Vital Events**

| During past 12 months | M | F |
|---|---|---|
| No. of births | | |
| No. of deaths | | |
| No. of abortions | | |
| No. of accidents | | |
| No. of pregnancies | | |
| No. of crimes/thefts | | |

## Causes of Disease/Death

| Sl. No. | Age | Sex | Cause of episode | Health care |
|---|---|---|---|---|
| | | | | |
| | | | | |
| | | | | |
| | | | | |
| | | | | |
| | | | | |
| | | | | |
| | | | | |
| | | | | |
| | | | | |
| | | | | |
| | | | | |
| | | | | |
| | | | | |
| | | | | |
| | | | | |
| | | | | |
| | | | | |
| | | | | |
| | | | | |
| | | | | |
| | | | | |
| | | | | |

**Source of health care preferred** : ____________________

Military hospital : ____________________

Private practitioners : ____________________

Civil hospital : ____________________

Self-care : ____________________

## GENERAL INFORMATION OF FAMILY MEMBERS

### (Persons Living in the Household)

| Sl. No. | Name | Relation with head of the family | Age | Sex | Marital | Status | Educational status | Occupation | Income | Present health status | Disability | Immunization | Health care taken | Remarks |
|---|---|---|---|---|---|---|---|---|---|---|---|---|---|---|
| | | | | | | | | | | | | | | |

A. General description of the members of the family not living in the household:
B. Eligible couples identified in the family:
C. Eligible couple practices Family planning Yes No
D. If yes, specify
E. If no, state reason

## Roles of Family Members

**Q. What are the assigned household tasks?**

**a. Adults**

**Male:** ____________________

____________________

**Female:** ____________________

____________________

**b. Children**

**Boys:** ____________________

____________________

____________________

**Girls:** ____________________

____________________

____________________

**Q. Relation of family members. How do they get along ?**

- Husband and wife ____________________
- Father and children ____________________
- Mother and children ____________________
- Children and children ____________________

**Q. Decision making in the family. Who makes the decision ?**

- Major decisions ____________________ (For example, hospitalization, family planning)
- Minor decisions ____________________ (For example, errands to market, collection of rations)

## COMPREHENSIVE FAMILY HEALTHCARE STUDY

### Antenatal and Postnatal Record

Name of the Mother: ____________________ Age: __________ Religion: ____________________

Husband's Name: ____________________ Age: __________ Occupation: ____________________

Address: ____________________

____________________

____________________

Gravida: __________ Para: __________ Date of LMP: __________ EDD: __________

### History of Previous Pregnancies

| Sl. No. | Age | Sex | FT/PM | Born alive/still-born | Living/dead | Healthy oth-erwise | Abortion in month | Pregnancy/NA | Labor/NA | Puerperium/NA |
|---|---|---|---|---|---|---|---|---|---|---|
| | | | | | | | | | | |

**Present Pregnancy**

| Date | Height of uterus | Position presentation | Head fixed/ floating | FHR/mt | Weight | Urine | | BP | HB | Investigations |
|---|---|---|---|---|---|---|---|---|---|---|
| | | | | | | Albumin | Sugar | | | |
| | | | | | | | | | | Blood VDRL<br><br>Height<br><br>Nutrition<br><br>Heart<br><br>Lungs<br><br>Breasts<br><br>Abdomen<br><br>Anemia<br><br>Edema<br><br>Vaginal discharge<br><br>Other abnormalities |

| Date | Treatment | Health teaching | Remarks | Signature |
|---|---|---|---|---|
| | | | | |

| Internal | | | | |
|---|---|---|---|---|
| Labor | Time | | | |
| | Date | Hours | Minutes | |
| Onset<br>Rupture of membranes<br>Birth of the child<br>Placenta<br>Total hours<br>Nature of delivery | | | | Membranes and placenta<br>Hemorrhage<br>Perineum-intact/lacerated<br>Episiotomy<br>Infant<br>Sex<br>Weight<br>Length<br>Head circumference<br>Condition at birth |

## Progress of the Mother—Postnatal

| Date | Temp | Pulse | Resp | Height of Uterus | Breasts | General condition and advice | Signature |
|---|---|---|---|---|---|---|---|
| | | | | | | | |

## Progress of the Child

| Date | Progress of the child | Signature |
|---|---|---|
| | | |

## Comprehensive Family Health Care Study

### Infant and Child Health Record

Name : ______________________
Sex : ______________________
Age : ______________________
Physical exam : ______________________

### If Normal, Mark 'O'; and If Abnormal, Mark 'X'

- Father's name: ______________________
- Mother's name: ______________________
- Address: ______________________
- Date of birth: __________ Birth weight: __________
- Birth history: ______________________ normal/abnormal
- Birth attendant: ______________________

| Month and Year | Weight (kg) | Height (cm) | Month and Year | Weight (kg) | Height (cm) |
|---|---|---|---|---|---|
| Jan<br>Feb<br>March<br>April<br>May<br>June | | | July<br>Aug<br>Sep<br>Oct<br>Nov<br>Dec | | |

**Immunizations**

| Name of vaccine | Date of immunization | | | | |
|---|---|---|---|---|---|
| BCG<br>DPT<br>TAB<br>Polio<br>TT<br>Cholera | | | | | |

**Development**

| | Yes | No |
|---|---|---|
| Head raised<br>Rolls over<br>Eruption of tooth<br>Sat with support<br>Without support<br>Sat alone walked with support<br>Talked<br>Walked alone<br>Bladder control<br>Bowel control | | |

| Physical exam. | If Normal, Mark 'O'; If Abnormal, Mark 'X' |
|---|---|
| Date<br>Age<br>Skin<br>Ears<br>Nose<br>Throat<br>Teeth and gum<br>Eyes<br>Bones<br>Joints<br>Liver<br>Spleen<br>Hb% | |
| **Dietery habits** | **Laboratory investigation** |
| | |

**Signs of Malnutrition (if observed mark)**

- Xerosis
- Bitot's spot
- Keratomalacia
- Dermatitis
- Glossitis
- Angular stomatitis
- Bow legs
- Edema
- Others (specify)

## Infectious Diseases

| | Age | Yes | No | Others (specify) | Age | Yes | No |
|---|---|---|---|---|---|---|---|
| Primary complex<br>Chicken pox<br>Measles<br>Whooping cough<br>Mumps | | | | | | | |

| Date | General health: Nutritional status, development and illness if any | Nurses observation, treatment and health teaching | Signature of CH nurse |
|---|---|---|---|
| | | | |

## School Health Service
## (Medical History Sheet)

Name of school: ____________________

Name of pupil: ____________________

Standard: ____________________

____________________

____________________

Age: __________ Years Sex: __________ M/F

Weight ________ kg Hight: ________ cms Chest: ________ cms Expansion: ______ cms.

General health and nutritional state

Protective inoculations: TAB/vaccination ____________________

Physical defects/Deformities: ____________________

CVS: ____________________

Respiratory system: ____________________

GI system: Teeth: ____________________

Gums: ____________________

Liver: ____________________

Spleen: ____________________

CNS: ____________________

Eyes: ____________________

Vision: RE ____________________

LE ____________________

Ears: RE ____________________

Hearing: LE ____________________

Special points: ____________________

____________________

____________________

____________________

____________________

____________________

**Signature of Medical Officer/Principal**

## Adults Health Card

Special points: ____________________

Name of head of family: ____________________

House No: ____________________

Village: ____________________ Sex: __________ Year of birth: __________

Name: ____________________

Marital status: ____________________

Education: ____________________

Occupation: ____________________

____________________

____________________

Income: ____________________

| Immunization date | Habits | | Post illness | |
|---|---|---|---|---|
| BCG | Betel leaves | ( ) | Tuberculosis | ( ) |
| TT | Tobacco | ( ) | STD | ( ) |
| TAB | Smoking | ( ) | Malaria | ( ) |
| Cholera | Alcohols | ( ) | Filaria | ( ) |
| Others | Others (specify) | ( ) | Dysentry | ( ) |

### Laboratory Investigations

| Date | Specimen findings | Treatment | Signature |
|---|---|---|---|
| | | | |

## Morbidity

| Date | Complaints | Positive findings | Diagnosis | Treatment | Advice follow-up | Signature |
|---|---|---|---|---|---|---|
| | | | | | | |

## Physical Health Assessment

Height: ________ cms. General health and Eyes vision LE RE

Weight: ________ kg. Nutritional status Ears hearing LE RE

Resp. system: Temp. P R

CNS:

Per abdomen: Liver: ______________ Spleen: ______________

Bowels and bladder function: Muscle skeletal system: Gait:

Mental and social health :

Adjustment aspects :

Family/work :

General outlook :

Hobbies interests :

Social circle :

Apparent physical/psychological defects

Special points:

# 14. PROJECT WORK

## ASSIGNMENT–32 (A): GROUP PROJECT

Conduct a group project—workshop, quiz, seminar, panel discussion and exhibition.
Write a lesson plan on the topic assigned to you.

Topic: __________

Project method: __________

Group: __________

Size of group: __________

Venue: __________

Date: __________

Time: __________ Venue: __________

Previous knowledge: __________

Method of teaching: __________

AV aids: __________

General objectives: __________

Specific objectives: __________

**Time specific objectives, content teaching and learning activities and AV aids evaluation**

**Summary**

**Bibliography**

# PROJECT WORK
## ASSIGNMENT–32 (B): GROUP PROJECT

Conduct a group project—workshop, quiz, seminar, panel discussion and exhibition.
Write a lesson plan on the topic assigned to you.

Topic: ____________________

Project method: ____________________

Group: ____________________

Size of group: ____________________

Venue: ____________________

Date: ____________________

Time: ____________________ Venue: ____________________

Previous knowledge: ____________________

Method of teaching: ____________________

AV aids: ____________________

General objectives: ____________________

Specific objectives:

**Time specific objectives, content teaching and learning activities and AV aids evaluation**

**Summary**

**Bibliography**

# PROJECT WORK
## ASSIGNMENT–32 (C): GROUP PROJECT

Conduct a group project—workshop, quiz, seminar, panel discussion and exhibition.
Write a lesson plan on the topic assigned to you.

Topic: ____________________

Project method: ____________________

Group: ____________________

Size of group: ____________________

Venue: ____________________

Date: ____________________

Time: ____________________ Venue: ____________________

Previous knowledge: ____________________

Method of teaching: ____________________

AV aids: ____________________

General objectives: ____________________

Specific objectives:

**Time specific objectives, content teaching and learning activities and AV aids evaluation**

**Summary**

**Bibliography**

# PROJECT WORK
## ASSIGNMENT–32 (D): GROUP PROJECT

Conduct a group project—workshop, quiz, seminar, panel discussion and exhibition.
Write a lesson plan on the topic assigned to you.

Topic: ______________________________

Project method: ______________________________

Group: ______________________________

Size of group: ______________________________

Venue: ______________________________

Date: ______________________________

Time: ____________________ Venue: ____________________

Previous knowledge: ______________________________

______________________________

______________________________

______________________________

______________________________

Method of teaching: ______________________________

______________________________

______________________________

______________________________

AV aids: ______________________________

______________________________

______________________________

General objectives: ______________________________

______________________________

______________________________

Specific objectives:

______________________________

______________________________

______________________________

______________________________

______________________________

______________________________

**Time specific objectives, content teaching learning activities and AV aids evaluation**

**Summary**

**Bibliography**

## PROJECT WORK
## ASSIGNMENT–32(E): GROUP PROJECT

Conduct a group project—workshop, quiz, seminar, panel discussion and exhibition.

Write a lesson plan on the topic assigned to you.

Topic: ______

Project method: ______

Group: ______

Size of group: ______

Venue: ______

Date: ______

Time: ______ Venue: ______

Previous knowledge: ______

Method of teaching: ______

AV aids: ______

General objectives: ______

Specific objectives:

**Time specific objectives, content teaching learning activities and AV aids evaluation**

**Summary**

**Bibliography**

## CERTIFIED BY

### Community Health Nursing

First year/second year/third year/fourth year

Class teacher ______________________________

Date: ____________________

____________________

Signature of seal of Principal

____________________

Signature
(Internal Examiner)

____________________

Signature
(External Examiner)

Date: ____________________

Date: ____________________

## REPEAT/SUPPLEMENTARY

### Community Health Nursing

First year/second year/third year/fourth year
Class teacher ______________________________

____________________

Signature
(Internal Examiner)

____________________

Signature
(External Examiner)

Date: ____________________

Date: ____________________

# BIBLIOGRAPHY


1. Basvanthappa BT. Community Health Nursing, 2nd Edition. New Delhi. Jaypee Brothers Medical Publication (P) Ltd 2008;pp.561-618.
2. Gulani KK. Community Health Nursing Principles and Practices, 1st Edition. Kumar Publishing House. 2005.
3. Gupta MC. Mahajan BK. Textbook of Preventive and Social Medicine, 3rd Edition. Jaypee Brothers Medical Publication (P) Ltd. 2007;pp.534-62.
4. Kasthuri Sundar. Community health nursing. 4th Edition. 2002;pp.574-604.
5. Kishores J. National health program of India, 7th Edition. Century Publication. 2007;pp.135-45.
6. Mohaja BK. Textbook of preventive and social medicine, 3rd Edition. Jaypee Brothers Medical Publishers, New Delhi. 2000.
7. Neerja KP. Textbook of sociology for nursing students. Jaypee Brothers Medical Publishers. 2006;pp. 526-38.
8. Park K. Park's. Textbook of preventive and social medicine, 19th Edition. Jabalpur. Banarsidas Bhanot Publisher. 2007.
9. Prabhakara GN. Textbook of community health for nurses, 1st Edition. India. PeeVee Pub. 2004.
10. Raj K. Women and development. Anmol Publication. 2000;pp.23-30.
11. Ram Ah. Social problem in India, 2nd Edition. Rivet Publication. 2006;pp.95-102.
12. Rao Sridhar. Community health nursing, 1st Edition. AITBS Publishers. 2006;pp.280-310.


## INTERNET


1. http://chiron.valdosta.edu/whuitt/col/behsys/psymtr.html
2. http://honolulu.hawaii.edu/intranet/committees/FacDevCom/guidebk/teachtip/domains.htm
3. http://tlt.its.psu.edu/suggestions/research/Psychomotor_Taxonomy.shtml